Bigger Than the Moon

SYREETA N. BROWN

Bigger Than the Moon

A Parent's Journey with Autism

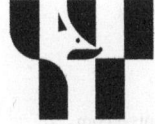

First published in 2025 by Syreeta N. Brown,
in partnership with Whitefox Publishing

www.wearewhitefox.com

Copyright © Syreeta N. Brown, 2025

Excerpt(s) from *The Bluest Eye* by Toni Morrison, copyright © 1970, copyright renewed 1998 by Toni Morrison. Used by permission of Alfred A. Knopf, an imprint of the Knopf Doubleday Publishing Group, a division of Penguin Random House LLC. All rights reserved.

Quote from *Polishing the Mirror* © 2013 by The Love Serve Remember Foundation, quote used with permission from the Publisher, Sounds True Inc.

Quote from *Everyday Tao* by Ming-Dao Deng. Copyright © 1996 By Deng Ming-Dao. Used by permission of HarperCollins Publishers.

Quote from *Collected Poems 1909-1962* by T.S. Eliot, copyright © 2002, used with permission from Faber and Faber Ltd.

ISBN 9781916797581
Also available as an eBook
ISBN 9781916797598

Syreeta N. Brown asserts the moral right to be identified as the author of this work.

All rights reserved. No part of this publication may be reproduced, stored in a retrieval system or transmitted in any form or by any means, electronic, mechanical, photocopying, recording or otherwise, without prior written permission of the author.

While every effort has been made to trace the owners of copyright material reproduced herein, the author would like to apologise for any omissions and will be pleased to incorporate missing acknowledgements in any future editions.

Designed and typeset by Couper Street Type Co.
Cover design by Anna Green
Cover images: girl by Muhammad_Zulfan/Shutterstock; moon by rawpixel.com
Project management by Whitefox

This book is dedicated to my son, Che, and to all the siblings of special needs children across the world – you are the true heroes. Che, I love you.

To all the Warrior Parents/Carers out there of children with special needs – know that you are never alone.

Contents

Prologue 1

The End 5
   Closing Door 7
   Day 1 – Hunter's Moon 17
   Falling Apart 46
   Metamorphosis 57
   The Middle 69
   Buffalo 76
   First Steps 88
   Discovery 97
   Mountains 115
   Descent 136
   Angels 140
   Bodhichitta 150
   Labalaba (Butterfly) 160
   Waxing Crescent 168

The Beginning 183
   Epilogue 196
   Lessons and Learning 199

Acknowledgements 203

What we call the beginning is often the end
And to make an end is to make a beginning.
The end is where we start from.

— T. S. ELIOT

There really is nothing more to say – except why. But since why is so difficult to handle, one must take refuge in how.

— TONI MORRISON

Prologue

I can hear the birds outside my bedroom window. I never heard them as much before as I do now. After everything that has happened this is the biggest point of note: the birds singing outside my bedroom window. They sound as if they are there for me, greeting the world in the morning with their call to action and seeing in the early evening with gentler tones. What is even more significant is that I would not have heard the birds five years before, given how much chaos was inside my world. The birds were always there; I just couldn't hear them.

I have not been able to admit any of this until now because I was in so much pain. Battling the end of my marriage whilst trying to maintain a sense of normality for my two children, managing my career through this and dealing with a diagnosis of autism for my daughter, Chloe.

I lost my inner voice. It fell silent and I turned inward with a resoluteness to survive and without many people that I could go to for help. Not because I had no one to help me but more I felt as if I would be admitting failure to ask them, unable to concede that I had got to a point in my life when I did not know what to do. Everything happened at once and it was as if I had been caught in the middle of something I could not explain, trapped with nowhere to turn or go.

I believe Chloe came into my life to take me from one level of living to a more enlightened place. It was a painful shift that triggered a transformation. This story of transformation focuses less on that awareness and more on the journey I have been on in that process. No doubt there are some reading this who have experienced that early stage of transition at the beginning of a major change but will not be able to recognise where I have found myself now because they are still stuck in that place where nothing can get in and there is no understanding of what is happening. That noiseless fog that consumes all your senses as you grapple to come to terms with what having a child diagnosed on the autistic spectrum means. I am writing for those who are in this place. For those of you who have reached the point I have now (with a lifetime still to go on this journey), this may still prove a useful read; a reminder that you are never alone and providing you with a shared sense of achievement that comes from knowing there are other parents out

Prologue

there, like you, struggling every day with this amazing but very challenging condition.

It's important to note that everyone's experience is different on this journey with autism. For those who just want to understand, I am hoping that the story of my journey creates more awareness of what being a parent of a child with autism can feel like. You may be a co-worker, a people manager, a friend or a family member of someone living with a child/children with autism. Either way, you have a critical role to play in the support that can be offered to those living with this condition as a part of their everyday lives. I write for those people, like me, who continue to work full-time and have the primary responsibility to keep the world turning for their families. It is a very lonely place to have a child diagnosed with a disability and not be surrounded every day with a systematic infrastructure that can help you; to have to fit into everything else the priority task of building the support for your child with very little space to be able to feel like you are doing this adequately and to piece together all the disparate sources, information, support and rules into some common thread that can help you build a plan for your child's needs.

My journey has been fraught with challenges but I can manage those challenges because of my determination to

Bigger Than the Moon

always have a plan for Chloe, in whatever way is required and however it needs to evolve and change. This is so she can be in the best possible position to fulfil her potential.

This is not a journal of medical references or information for you to deconstruct and decipher and compare to your own situation. My aim is to tell my story of the world that surrounded me as I embarked on this journey with Chloe, and to focus on how I managed the impact of diagnosis, along with other elements of my life. I share what I've learnt, so far, in forging a way forward for Chloe, her brother and myself: many of the steps were not planned but learnt, and some were discovered through the experience of others. I hope that the words that follow can provide those in a similar situation with some help, comfort and perhaps guidance, as you embark on your own journey to build the plan for your child.

The End

Closing Door

After a difficult pregnancy and dramatic birth, Chloe was born. The pregnancy had not been normal, and from the beginning I felt as if this was going to be very different from the experience of having my first child.

The story of Chloe's arrival into the world is very important in understanding what I went through and how it helped me later on when she was initially diagnosed with autism.

I instinctively knew something was wrong when I fell pregnant with Chloe. It was a feeling of unsettledness I could not shake. From the moment I did the pregnancy test it was not how I expected to feel. I went through the early stage of pregnancy with awful morning sickness that beat my previous pregnancy by a mile. What had also been clear to me was the rapid growth of my stomach. By the fourth month of pregnancy my stomach looked more like five/six months and it felt uncomfortable in parts and more than just the swelling associated with pregnancy. I ended up being diagnosed with polyhydramnios, which

Bigger Than the Moon

is the medical term for excess fluid in the amniotic sac. Something was happening to me and I could not explain or articulate this to anyone. During bouts of severe morning sickness, that could actually occur at any point during the day, I was confronted by an all-consuming sensation of being emptied of something, as if I was being jolted out of my present state of awareness into something else. The projectile vomiting was, quite simply, horrific, almost violent, as if I was being shaken mentally as well as physically. I could not believe that pregnancy alone had created this state of disruption in me. It was like the feeling you have when waking from a nightmare that you can't remember; the physical sensation is there but your mind is not quite able to recollect the exact nature of the dream that created that feeling in the first place. This was how I felt each day and every time I was sick.

At my twenty-week scan I knew that I was carrying a girl before they told me. I could tell just by looking at the image on the screen and felt an immediate emotional connection to her. It was something I could not explain. Chloe was not a big mover or kicker, however, and this was always a question of concern for me, although those concerns were always abated with reassurance from the medical professionals that any movement, however limited, was a good sign. My son, Che, had performed acrobatics in my stomach, and so I was not used to this feeling of scheduled but very limited movements. I voiced my concerns and when a second scan had to be performed because Chloe had not moved enough for them to see all the critical organs, they identified the polyhydramnios, which meant that I had to be regularly monitored to observe the levels on a bi-weekly basis. My stomach continued to grow at pace and reflected a much later stage of pregnancy. The pressure began to take its toll on my abs, with a sensation like physical snaps of my abdominal muscles occurring at moments when I was trying to move my body up to stand from a seated position and from one side to another – in fact anything that required the use of my stomach muscles. My pelvic floor became severely affected from the increasing burden of weight, making walking very painful and difficult. By 31 weeks, and with a stomach that looked more like 40 weeks, I had begun to feel the very mild contractions that can happen with polyhydramnios pregnancies. Throughout all of this I was working full-time as a Head of HR in a large FTSE 100 organisation and caring for my son. In my role I had responsibility for a team of HR professionals and led the People Strategy for a business unit of around 7,000 people. It was interesting and challenging work, which was exactly what I liked.

Bigger Than the Moon

I had been a working parent by this point for around five years and had got used to the daily juggle of balancing work with my parenting duties, nursery drop-offs and pickups. It was hard work, and now with my pregnancy became even more so. It was always important to me that I would be as present in my son's life as I was meeting my work commitments, so the strain of a difficult pregnancy began to add to the increasing feelings of guilt that I had been battling with as a working parent. Che was a happy child and innocently unaware of the military-like system that enabled his happiness and active schedule! His dad and I worked together to ensure his schedule was the priority. My company offered a flexible working policy that accommodated home working, so I would travel into the office for meetings as well as being able to work in person with my team and engage with my business partners. I was grateful that given the increasing physical and emotional burden of pregnancy I did not have to commute every day.

By 32 weeks, however, exhausted by being superwoman, I calmly phoned the labour ward as I had begun to feel slight but persistent contractions. They told me to come straight in and I arrived at the hospital almost in a daze and ready for whatever was to happen next. After a few hours of observations, they admitted me for one week to halt the onset of labour and put me on complete bed rest. I then came home and was told I could not go back to work in the office and that doing any form of physical activity, even walking, would be potentially dangerous. I was told it could trigger the onset of labour, which could result in the collapse of the umbilical cord if my waters broke suddenly because of the level of fluids in the amniotic sac. In a moment my world had dramatically shifted from busy productive days to a stillness that seemed alien to me. I had gone from commuting and juggling diaries and meetings to silent days, only broken up by the routine of Che going to school and then coming home.

It was during this period that my little baby and I began to build a strong bond – we only had each other for company most of the day and a very set routine. I would struggle to get up and showered. I got dressed slowly and would go downstairs and seat myself in the same spot on the sofa that had an indentation from the regularity of the process! Che would be running around like any boisterous five-year-old getting ready for school and would leave with his dad. I then planned the day, which consisted of watching movies, with regular breaks for food. The anticipation of food would be preceded by a bit of movement from the small body inside mine. Once the food was digested her hiccups would begin, yet I was still unnerved by the

Bigger Than the Moon

lack of significant movement and watched every day for signs that she was still alive and healthy.

I had been given the option of a caesarean but my real fear of operations and anaesthesia meant that I remained resolute that Chloe would be delivered naturally. At just approaching 37 weeks I could bear the weight and pain no longer and elected to be induced. It was a real moment of giving in and surrendering to something that I knew I had no control over. Chloe's birth was like the arrival of a storm; one that begins almost gently with mild rain showers but quickly increases in intensity and force, ending with thunder and lightning. At the beginning, I had slight contractions and discomfort, all bearable, but building with strength as the hours went by. A shift came after five hours but rather than a gradual move into the intensity of final labour pain, it was like an instant change in pain level. By this time painkillers were not an option and I was forced to endure two more hours of some of the most intense contractions and pain ever. Unlike my first experience of labour, there was no build up and gradual progression; I felt as if I had been in full control of that experience. This was completely different. I had lost all control, as if the process was taking me over and I could not connect my mind with my body; something I had been so proud of achieving in my first delivery with

Closing Door

my son, benefitting from well-practised yogic breathing. With the arrival of Chloe there was no room for breathing – more like gasping for air! I wanted to feel as if I was in control but this proved impossible and I could not understand why. It honestly felt like someone else had taken over, and I had been unceremoniously dethroned from the role of giving birth. At one point, delirious and dehydrated, I was put on a drip which I ripped out of my arm from the force of raising my arms to alleviate the pain and reaching for some imaginary relief in the air. I was defeated in my aim to understand and control what was happening. The battle had been lost and so was I, in this room with just the midwives in front of me and Chloe's father beside me. I remember that as quickly as the storm had arrived, it left and then all around me became silent. I could not hear a thing in spite of their voices encouraging me and my own voice coming out in rasps of air and gasps. It was as if my body had become separated from my consciousness. Everything became distant.

Chloe came out with such force, as if signalling to the world that something very important had happened. Her arrival was followed by a very unnerving silence. She was not breathing as the cord had been tightly wrapped around her neck, which had been the fear for a natural delivery with a polyhydramnios pregnancy. They removed it very quickly but spent a couple of minutes, which felt like hours, getting her to breathe. Everyone remained calm but I knew something was wrong. I was too exhausted to look over and just overwhelmed with relief that the process I had just gone through was over. Eventually she cried and I began to relax. I reflect often on that moment and wonder if things would have been different for Chloe if I had elected for the caesarean. There are so many 'ifs' and 'buts' around Chloe's autism. I try not to think too hard about choices made and decisions reached; they won't change things for her now. I will leave those ifs and buts for the researchers. Now and again, however, the feeling of responsibility will overwhelm me and make me sad for a moment. Then I remember I am human and forgive myself for thinking too much.

Chloe was born and life stopped, for a while at least. There was an unease, for me, in everything, which was triggered from the anxiety around Chloe's birth and a feeling that I had lost complete control of my life at that moment. Looking back, I can see now that a door was closing on one phase of my life and I was slowly walking towards another one. It was as if Chloe being born moved me into a new place in life. Everything changed from her birth.

Initially this was reflected in the fact that I could not move – literally. I was very reliant on the support of

Closing Door

Chloe's dad during this time for almost everything, which was an unusual situation for me to be in given my love of independence and always being quite self-reliant. I was uncomfortable with this feeling of dependence, which is how I saw it during this time. However, we continued to work as parents together in spite of the unspoken personal distance that was becoming more apparent. I had gone from multi-tasking, commuting, back-to-back meetings, conference calls, managing a large team and running around after Che, to a complete stop. My pelvic floor was so painful, and this made it almost impossible to walk, even for a few steps. The impact and burden of the excess fluid that I had been forced to carry around for the last nine months had taken its toll. After the birth, I struggled to breathe and became out of breath very quickly with even the slightest movement. I had to physically pause at each step before I could move any further. I had also developed a hernia whilst pregnant with Chloe that became very apparent and obtrusive once she left my womb. It bobbled around, as if to remind me of the presence of her that had once been there. I was mortified. It felt like I was having an out-of-body experience. Everything about this pregnancy, the labour and after-effects, felt wrong. I just felt it and did not express this to anybody. This was a deliberate choice as I had retreated into myself after

Bigger Than the Moon

Chloe was born and I had started to become disengaged with many people around me.

I felt increasingly isolated in the early days of Chloe's life – more of an emotional isolation than physical. I still maintained a regular pattern in some respects as Che provided me with an anchor and both his dad and I got on with the normal routine of life as much as my physical condition allowed, but I sensed things were changing.

Day 1 – Hunter's Moon

Chloe had never moved much in my stomach and after she was born that stillness continued. Once she joined me in this external world, the first thing I observed was that she had a distinct way of looking around at her environment, almost as if she had been here before and was recollecting things. It was uncanny and I was fascinated, watching her for hours. She was not one of those babies that wriggled around a lot and she did not actually make much noise. She was an observer who only made a sound if unexpectedly disturbed. People would often tell me how 'good' she was. I realised how much I was solely focused on her as a result of all the things I was discovering about Chloe even in those early days. My whole attention became absorbed by her, and my curiosity went beyond that of a new mother learning about her newborn child. The same period with Che was not as intense in terms of my observation

Bigger Than the Moon

of him but was more about me learning how to be a parent and worrying if I was doing the right things or making mistakes. With Chloe, it was more about how different I felt she was and being very curious about that. I remember taking her home from the hospital. I dressed her slowly and positioned her carefully in the car seat. The hernia that seemed to have replaced her presence in my womb continued to keep me focused on what had just happened and slowed me down somewhat. Chloe looked at me enquiringly almost as if to say, 'Where are we going?' She had a frown on her face but did not make a sound. I always remember how she looked at me deeply – and she still has that look to this day. I know what it means now: she was silently trying to figure out what was going on, like her mind and brain were trying to connect things. At that time half of me thought it was just the behaviour of a newborn infant and the other half of me wondered. Che had been less observant as a newborn, pretty nondescript and sleepy, as most babies are, only seeming alert and requiring attention when he wanted to be fed.

I found Chloe fascinatingly alert and bright, and as we walked over to the car I saw that she seemed unfazed by the external environment and still did not make a sound. The only thing that made her jump was the sudden loud

Day 1 – Hunter's Moon

noise of a horn nearby. As her car seat got fixed by her dad, I got in the car beside her, and I remember letting out a big sigh. It had taken all of the little energy I had left to make the journey from the hospital room to the car. Everything was so much slower now in my life and I was not used to it. I struggled with this sense of time coming to a halt, as if everything continued to move around me but I had stopped. I would find out later that this was an important place to be when trying to figure Chloe out. At this point, however, I just felt impatient and unclear with this space where I found myself: in between what had happened and what was ahead.

When we arrived home that first day – as a family of four now – my sister had prepared a sweet welcome home and put pink balloons up. They bobbed up and down with the force of the warm air rising from the heating that was on: it was early October and although the sun was shining the air had started to get that crisp chill to it. I remember looking at the balloons and thinking of my hernia making the same movement in my stomach. The moment felt bittersweet. I wanted to be happy but I felt exhausted and weary. Not just from the physical experience of giving birth but I still felt something was not right. I sat on the sofa and looked at Chloe in her car seat on the living-room floor and wondered what was next.

Bigger Than the Moon

Che was introduced to his sister in hospital. He looked at her both with the curiosity of a five-year-old and bemusement of a newly made sibling. He stared at her and she stared back. He kept a cautious distance, however, safe enough to look without having to touch her. This moment was the beginning of a beautiful relationship. In all the challenges that I would face going forward, there was never any doubt in my mind that he would always love and protect her. I knew she was a special baby before she was identified with special needs and in his own way I think Che did too, which is even more of a reason why he became so close to her. When she arrived home, if there was a small moment where I may not have been within sight of her, or even if I was, he would be quick to tell me if she had started to make a noise, would ensure her blanket remained in place if she started to move in a way that disrupted its angle over her body and talked to her as if she could understand everything he was saying. He observed her as much as I did and was seriously attentive. She adored him and her first smile was for him.

However, for me the birth of Chloe had triggered the buried memory of long-held beliefs around the early days of motherhood I had experienced with Che, and I

Day 1 – Hunter's Moon

became even more lost in the idea that everything was falling apart. I felt inadequate as a mother and had a sense that I had never mastered the perceived 'skill' that I thought motherhood was with my son when he was a baby. At the time I did not recognise that this was a myth and parenting is a process of learning, with some things coming easily and others taking time to develop. Looking back on his arrival and this initial experience of motherhood, I now realise I had been experiencing postnatal depression but this was not acknowledged at the time either by myself or those around me, for I was the person who everyone looked to for the answer. I was always in control and sure of where I was going and a high achiever. The moment of becoming a mother challenged that idea about who I was; it had now become a burden in many ways. I realised that I was not in control and for the first time wanted help to navigate this new path. But instead of being able to voice these needs, I blamed myself for feeling that way, and as a result of that, I felt like I was somehow taking back control because it was down to me. I had felt so capable with everything in my life up until motherhood.

My children's father came from a big family, and he seemed to be far more adept at parenting than me, or so I thought at the time based on the traditional idea I had of

Bigger Than the Moon

'parenting'. His dad appeared comfortable with managing what I felt was Che's constant crying and unsettledness as he went through a period of being affected by colic. Observing his ease made my feelings of inadequacy grow. As a baby, I believe my son sensed my feelings and so clung to his father's confidence and would only settle and be calmed by him. Che's crying was an incessant reminder of the new skill I seemed unable to master, and so I would often yield him to his father's embrace and care, much as I loved him and longed to be clung to as well. In spite of this I was a diligent mother who adored her son and learnt to care for him in a way that got stronger over time rather than making the immediate connection that some mothers have with their newborns. Eventually I realised that this is a common experience of new mothers.

When Chloe arrived, however, I was determined to connect and do things differently and fight any feelings of depression that I thought may overcome me. I was completely focused on observing her, and to an extent forgot about myself and how I felt. In a funny kind of way this helped me navigate the feelings I had, be that the pain of physical recovery or the sadness that would come over me in waves. Because of this intense focus, I believe I saw signs very early in her development that things were not as they should be. It was as if I was still in a state of

Day 1 – Hunter's Moon

heightened alert, continuing from the early days of my pregnancy when things just did not feel right.

Chloe's journey into the medical world commenced with the results of her heel prick test given to newborn infants to test for certain hereditary conditions. Her results came back positive for sickle cell trait. As a trait, there was no risk of her developing the conditions associated with sickle cell, but in the event that Chloe was to meet a partner with a trait then their children, should they have any, would have a very high chance of being born with sickle cell anaemia. The interesting thing was that when I read the letter, rather than feel relieved, I had this sense that it would be the beginning of a very long journey with Chloe. This was all intuitively felt, however, and I never expressed it outwardly to anyone.

For the first couple of months, Chloe's life was very simple, albeit she was surrounded by huge transformation. The US had a real chance of electing its first Black president in Barack Obama and during October the news was filled with the final leg of dramatic campaigning. I would be stationed in my bedroom with Chloe in my arms, watching the television on the wall, mesmerised by the change that was taking place in America. In some ways this moment reflected the feelings of change that were taking place in my life, although this was on a much smaller scale in comparison to world events, but huge for me all the same.

My world became very small and intense. I realised that everything I had been and all the things I thought my life was about were being challenged. It felt as if I was being forced to create an opening to something else. But for a while as the door seemed to close on the way things were, I didn't look to see where things may be going. For a while, I stayed married and pretended that everything was okay and that it would work out. For a while, I carried on smiling at the school gates with the other parents and forcing a sense of normality into my life that I knew was a lie. In this unclear place, I drowned myself in Chloe as I felt safe with her and sure of what my role was: I clung to her with all my heart. She was breast-feeding well (something I had struggled to do effectively with Che) and I was determined that this would continue for the next four months before I would face the inevitable weaning required so that I could go back to work when she reached six months. I felt positive in the way I was connecting with Chloe and felt confident around her in spite of the uncertainty I felt around her development.

From a very early stage Chloe grounded me and gave me purpose, which would be an important thing as I went through the journey with her. These moments were

Day 1 – Hunter's Moon

probably the quietest and most peaceful of the journey Chloe and I have had together in life so far. Nothing dramatic happened during the day and we created a routine around Che's school start and end times as well as catching up with friends, when I could.

Something happened, however, that started the journey into isolation for me that was to continue all the way through to Chloe's diagnosis and the couple of years afterwards. Chloe began to break out in eczema on her face, arms and chest. It was mild at first, appearing as a subtle rash, and at one point I even put it down to the 'milk' spots babies get in those early days. But it rapidly started to deteriorate into something much worse. Her skin started to get extremely sore and red, eventually becoming infected. It was so hard to watch her get irritated at such a small age and be in discomfort. The sores were horrendous and I felt helpless as her skin condition deteriorated, so much so that it proved to be the beginning of her journey into the medical world of observations, blood tests, creams, treatments and antibiotics and numerous referrals to specialists. It had begun: she was just three months old.

A letter dated 6 January 2009 from Chloe's consultant dermatologist, Dr Manning, details her diagnosis of 'infected atopic eczema'. It outlines that she has been prescribed an oral antibiotic and was given Fucidin cream. It lists the endless other creams she has had up until that point to try to address and halt the rapid progress of the eczema: Aveeno cream, Epaderm and Oilatum gel.

She also had to have blood tests taken for the first time to test for certain genetic conditions that may have been contributing towards the cause of her eczema. I had to take her to our local NHS hospital. She lay on the bed and the nurses were amazing with her and she displayed the braveness (or blissful ignorance!) that was to become her trademark as well as her beaming smile that melted a thousand hearts. I remember the nurses putting cream on her skin to numb the area and then, before she realised, it was over and as she considered whether to commence crying, she looked up at my smiling, confident face reassuring her, and paused to consider her next move and then smiled back. Chloe smiled with her eyes. They held so much beauty in those tiny spaces, which suggested a whole world inside. My heart was always moved by her smile.

The tests detailed that most things were normal but she had a very low level of zinc. She was subsequently prescribed a zinc supplement. I would later discover significant research around the link of zinc deficiency to autism, but at this point I was just trying to manage and

Day 1 – Hunter's Moon

understand what was happening with my little baby who seemed so vulnerable and delicate at this early stage of her life and in so much discomfort.

During this time, whilst Chloe's father and I began to drift apart in terms of our marriage, we became closer in another way as a result of focusing our energies on her, almost like football fans at a game or people watching the match together in the pub who are complete strangers, until they celebrate a goal scored by their team. At this point my world was so painful. I was a spinning mess: thinking about Chloe, worried about whether I was being present enough for my little son, panicking about returning to work in three months. I was also still feeling physically weak from the pregnancy and birth. Most of all I felt alone, knowing that my marriage was breaking down and not being able to tell a soul.

One particular night in what had become a familiar scene I was upstairs alone with Chloe, whilst her dad was downstairs with our son. Chloe was having great difficulty breathing. I called down to him as I was starting to get concerned. We recognised the familiar heavy chest movements that appeared to suggest asthma; our son was a sufferer and both Chloe's dad and my brother had also been chronic asthmatics. On top of everything else I was distraught. She was still so tiny and it felt like everything

Bigger Than the Moon

was happening to her. We quickly got her dressed and rushed to A&E. I remember sitting in the car quietly after strapping her into the car seat at the back. Ever since Chloe had been born, and with all the events that were surrounding me, I was on a constant state of high alert, feeling a sense of panic and nervousness, waiting for the next drama to unfold, even if things were pretty normal. I realise now that this is a typical symptom of anxiety and was being brought about by a succession of things that seemed to be happening to me all at once. I was completely overwhelmed.

My heart was racing as we drove to the hospital with our son in tow, who didn't seem too disturbed by this unexpected trip to the hospital. It was fairly late, so the A&E reception area seemed empty, and given Chloe's age and condition she was prioritised for triage to assess what may be wrong. I will never forget the young junior doctor who came into the small room, lit very brightly by the fluorescent lighting in the ceiling. She seemed young and relatively new to her work and immediately set upon a thorough examination of Chloe. As she took her stethoscope to Chloe's chest I could see Chloe's stomach cavity moving deeply in and out like someone was pumping air inside her. She was such a good baby and at no time did she make a sound, she just looked up at

Day 1 – Hunter's Moon

me with imploring eyes that seemed to say 'Help me'. I would see this look often over the years. After a while I started to get concerned as I could see the doctor was trying to identify something that seemed more than just confirming my initial prognosis that Chloe was having some form of asthma attack triggered by a chest infection. She looked up at both of us with her hand still trained on the stethoscope, holding it firmly on Chloe's chest, and quietly asked us, 'Has Chloe ever been diagnosed with a heart condition?'

We looked at her and then at each other and simultaneously said 'No' with a tone of complete surprise. She continued in a non-committal way but still serious enough to warrant our attention, 'I am not sure but it feels like I can hear a murmur of some sort but it will need some further investigation from a specialist.' She closed the statement with confirmation of what I had initially suspected, that Chloe had a chest infection that had caused asthma-like symptoms and she would be issued with the standard antibiotics (again).

I was impressed with the doctor's insightful knowledge, being open to more than just the symptom she was observing and her commitment to being thorough. I found this experience was becoming increasingly rare in a system that was suffering (and continues to suffer) from setbacks and cutbacks and a lack of time for doctors to do anything more than just what was required. I had initially perceived her youth to be inexperience, but whilst she may have been fairly new to her profession, she demonstrated the power of curiosity coupled with ability and potential; a trait I had recognised often in the work I did in Human Resources as being the hallmark of talented people who would progress. Her insight that evening, and the events that it triggered shortly after, was the thing that would help us understand more about Chloe's health that we may not have discovered at such an early stage of her life.

Chloe was provided with a nebuliser at the hospital and observed for a couple of hours and then we were told that she could go home but a referral letter would need to be sent to a heart specialist. Fortunately, because of the benefits package I had at work, I had access to private healthcare insurance, so I could organise this relatively quickly with my local GP.

As a full-time working mother I was often plagued with the guilt-ridden feelings about how inadequate I was in any one part of my life, never feeling like I was being completely effective in any of it, even though the opposite was true. However, there would be many moments like this where I would appreciate the access I had to the support available from my employer. In some ways, this

Day 1 – Hunter's Moon

created a dependency with my employer which for me was a positive; however, it did make me reflect how frustrating it must be for parents who don't have that option, and the choice. Getting quick access to the right care and support for your child should happen in an equitable way regardless of your employment status and financial means, and sadly this is not always the case in our current system.

We got Chloe home and as usual with both my kids when they were sick, I slept half-awake, constantly checking that she was breathing. I made an appointment for the GP the next day and got my letter for the consultant who we would go and see the following week.

I had decided to drive up to the clinic in central London given my increasing awareness of Chloe's skin condition and how people would stare, which had started to make me feel uncomfortable. Being slow and still in pain also made it difficult for me to navigate the buggy and newborn baby on public transport. Once I arrived on the street where the clinic was, I had the task of finding a parking bay. I remember stopping for a while in the car and looking out through the front windscreen. It was raining and although it was hitting the screen lightly it was almost as if I could not hear it, just see it. Everything was silent to me in the outside world and inside of me was a loud noise that could

Bigger Than the Moon

not come out. I was exhausted and sad. I felt like I was failing again in this world of motherhood as I could not make things better for my baby girl. I remember starting to feel a tear come out of each eye and I quickly pulled myself together and held it all in instinctively in my effort to try to gain that sense of control that I craved. I would do that often over the next few years.

I stepped out into the rain, not caring much for how it was making me appear, just focused on protecting Chloe from the cold rain and wind. I opened the back passenger door of the car and she looked up at me, reassured to see my face, and I felt a little better, remembering I was here to help her. So I quickly moved into action. I walked the few steps to the entrance, struggling with rain, baby bag and the weight of the car seat, and rang the buzzer. The door opened and I pushed with the side of my body whilst holding on to her car seat with both hands. This upper body strength would be a necessity as Chloe grew older; little did I know that all these things were preparation for the journey.

As we waited I remember looking around the clinic. Its furnishings and artwork cleverly created a sense of calm and reinforced the ease with which the receptionist greeted me and guided me through the paperwork. Everything was effortless.

Day 1 – Hunter's Moon

We were shown to the consultant's office. Dr Davis was to become a familiar face to Chloe and me. Whilst the space he occupied in the basement of this well-presented establishment felt a little opulent, he had a down-to-earth style that disarmed me; so much so that I cantered through telling the story of Chloe's first four months of life with efficacy and speed. I could tell he was impressed with my ability to recount everything that had happened and the events that had led to me seeing him. He listened attentively and said that he would need to perform a physical examination and an echocardiogram. I looked at Chloe's tiny four-month-old body and felt slightly scared as she was quite a mover by this stage and needed to be extremely still in order for the echocardiogram to work. He reassured me and I undressed Chloe to her nappy and looked at her with a smile. She smiled back. Dr Davis had the same calming effect on Chloe. I had noted that Chloe became very still when she found herself in different environments and took the time to look around and see where she was, sometimes looking a little anxious. She also became entranced by different lighting. As Dr Davis dimmed the lighting, the neon shapes of figures meant to distract children and keep them amused had a fascinating effect on Chloe. She was very focused on the different colours suddenly appearing in the darkened room. After

Bigger Than the Moon

the echocardiogram was performed she also had an ECG, which took the form of sticking tiny electrodes on to her body. It felt like it took ages but it was maybe fifteen to twenty minutes altogether. Chloe had remained as still as could be expected but it was enough for a diagnosis to be made. She had in fact been born with a small hole in the heart. Medically speaking, a Ventricular Septal Defect (VSD). It was small enough that he felt there was no need for medical intervention at this stage, but she would need to be observed periodically to assess whether it was closing and if any further treatment or medical intervention was required.

I remember thinking a few years later, as I reflected on this time, how appropriate it was that this little girl, my angel, had been born with a small hole in her heart. That one of the most vital organs in her body, which I believe connects the physical body with the soul, was somehow not ready to complete its formation at exactly the same time that I had my heart broken in so many ways. She was effectively born with a broken heart but it was working hard to heal itself. From this point on she and I were officially soulmates.

I kept the drawing that Dr Davis did at the time on his clinic headed paper. I remember him taking out an elegant fountain pen and he drew a normal heart and then

Day 1 – Hunter's Moon

a picture of one with a VSD, all the time explaining to me what I was seeing, how the condition worked, and how her heart could potentially heal itself. He wrote his name and contact details and we were to see him periodically over the next couple of years to review the development of her condition.

7 March 2006 (journal note of a creative writing piece as part of a short story course)

Italy, Lake Maggiore
Grandmother died today, and with her all the answers to questions never asked. The image of her grasping for life is etched in my mind like the scraping of chalk on a blackboard. Despite the traumatic and violent picture of her fighting an enemy who had already won, the thing that stands out the most the last time I saw her was the pitiful state of her fingers. I had always held a fond regard for my grandmother's hands; they told a story so gracefully, without her needing to utter one single word. Long and elegant, they were perfectly manicured and as you entered

Bigger Than the Moon

the room you would be instantly drawn to these worthy hosts. They beckoned you in and you envied them quietly, like a guest who knew they did not belong in the presence of such superior beauty. Her fingers were the one part of her that I could reach and feel. All other areas were hidden from view and her soul a secret she would never reveal. Her eyes were the only part that hinted what lay beneath this surface of superior calm and even then, there was a coldness that refused to break. In that last visit at the hospital they looked tired and old, almost shrinking away from sight, perhaps curled in pain.

Even now, I can see her in my mind's eye; wretched as the pain of the illness takes hold and rapidly spreads through her body, like bamboo leaves adorning a deserted garden. She holds me with her stare and moves her mouth. I stare back and the two of us remain defiant; one refusing to give in to the other.

'Come over here – I need something.' She stares and fixes her glare at me. I silently stare back and fix my gaze on her like a needle on skin.

She closes her eyes and I am frozen, wondering if this is it. Will this be the moment that death

Day 1 – Hunter's Moon

arrives? But the silence is shattered by her gasping breath and she opens her dry and contorted mouth to speak.

She told me to get her some water. I was shocked as the starkness of her impolite voice hit me, like shattered glass that had been blown, by the force of the blast, against my skin. What I wanted to hear I did not – instead her determination, even whilst dying, to appear in control continued. She was almost presidential, as she assumed the upper hand in this silent battle that we had commenced.

I am reflecting on this last moment as I walk past the mountains of the Alps. They are beaming majestically over the beautiful Italian Lake Maggiore and I wonder if she is with me right now. It is almost as if I feel her presence still refusing to leave. I imagine that heaven is asking her questions so she can gain permission to walk through, and enter a new realm of existence. I wonder if she will make it.

A voice behind me disturbed me from my thoughts.

It was Jessica, a fellow student on this business course I decided to continue with, even though

Bigger Than the Moon

I had been told my grandmother did not have long to live. I responded to Jessica mechanically and smiled as we continued walking. She knew my grandmother had died and there existed that silence that lingers when there is nothing that can be said. We continued walking and a boat moved past on the calm water, against the immovable and dominant presence of the mountains. Spring was arriving and the snow caps had started to disappear as nature intended. The only thing I was certain of at that very moment was that winter was ending. I moved into my coat and folded my arms to keep out the chill that had overcome me. I was somewhere nobody knew me. The feeling of being lost and anonymous was almost comforting. We made our way over the pier.

I sat down and watched all kinds of people walk by on the pathways next to the lake and my eyes wandered over their moving figures and were drawn to a distant island in the middle. It was perfectly cultivated with a castle regally positioned at the centre. I was captivated by this magnificent sight and wondered how something so beautiful and enchanting could be so alone

Day 1 – Hunter's Moon

in the middle of the grand lake. I made a mental note to go over and visit the island.

I recalled just before arriving here to this beautiful part of Italy, how alone I thought my grandmother was in her hospital ward despite sharing what can only be described as a corridor with four other people. Her curtains were drawn, even though the nurses had insisted they remain open. It was cold in the ward and I remember watching her sleeping, but not peacefully. Her eyes were closed but her lids flicked, betraying the movement beneath them that was clearly taking place; she appeared to be waging a battle. I knew this because her body moved suddenly now and again as if the pain urged her to move to the next life, but she was holding firm. As I watched her I thought of the past and how powerful it had been in the story of this woman's life, yet she refused to fully allow it to surface and breathe, hiding it away and creating a barrier for those around her.

I recalled a few months before this cold and empty scene at the hospital. She was moving slowly in a small room that was always the coldest in the house. It was January and the chill of the

Bigger Than the Moon

winter seemed to penetrate every part of the house, but nowhere as much as in this room. She was slower than normal, gently carrying her small yet tall frame and still managing to appear graceful despite her ageing body indicating otherwise. Her hands like feathers fell swiftly on a box and she opened it with a quiet urgency and looked up at me as if to signal that something important was about to commence. I was silent but acknowledged this solemn occasion with reverence and looked back at her intently. I knew this was important for my grandmother, but she remained calm, almost indifferent as she always did. As the lid of the box opened, a mirror-like object came into view, slowly, but with a flash of light into my face, reflected from the only window in the room that had the sun's rays pushing through it. At that moment, it seemed as if the doors of heaven had opened in the small, dark room and she smiled. She appeared to remember something from that deeply hidden part of her life and turned to look at me. I remember she said that she wanted me to have the object that was in her hands.

There was no softness in her voice; just a confidence that seemed to indicate that this

Day 1 – Hunter's Moon

would mean something to me. She continued, her memory clearly transported to somewhere else and said to me: 'My beautiful blue dress. It was silk,' and she paused before continuing with a sigh in her patois, tinged with a tone of American, 'and the colour – the colour was blue... different, you know?'

I remember moving my stare from her face to the object that had now come into view. She turned it away from the light at the window. It was her wedding picture, but not your typical wedding photo: a frame that was a glass mirror, with her placed at its centre: the frame was a typical style that graced the walls of many Caribbean families in the 60s and 70s in London. She is sitting on a stool, with her head facing to the front and her body at an angle to the side, in a 60s-style sky-blue knee-length gown. Her hands are placed regally on her lap and one is placed in its white glove. The other is without the glove and has her wedding ring clearly visible. There is no groom, however, just her. She is staring into the lens intently, almost defiant, as if in a state of victory. I notice that she is not smiling. I did not understand why that picture,

Bigger Than the Moon

of all the pictures in her house, was the one she chose to give to me.

I think of that moment as I remembered staring at her lying in the hospital bed with her jerking body movements – still fighting and I wanted her to let go but could tell she would not. Her feet were in my hands and I embraced them, gently rubbing the soles to help soothe her, thinking that somehow I could rub away the disease that at this very moment was ravaging her entire body.

She looked at me and smiled, and quietly moved her mouth as sound whispered out through her lips, husky but reassuring,

'Yes, that is good – over there – take the balm.' She painfully and slowly lifted her arm to point to the tiger balm on the table and I picked it up.

There was no noise on the ward now, just us. I took the balm and slowly unscrewed the lid. The aroma of menthol hit my face like a gust of wind announcing an arrival. I took some in my hand and moved it over her feet. They were fragile in my hands and I held her feet with care and started to massage rhythmically and deliberately. She closed her eyes. I saw a tired body through

Day 1 – Hunter's Moon

her defiance and resistance, but a soul fighting to live. I realised that my relationship with her was like a tug of war between love and hate – whose pull was constant but favoured no sides. It was magnetic but without a lasting attachment. It was neither beautiful nor ugly. I sometimes loathed her indifference, even despised her, and at other times felt a deep sense of respect, love and admiration for her beauty, strength and resilience. It was a conflicting type of love and one I did not fully understand. Not back then anyway. My love for my mother meant that as a result I struggled to completely love her mother: I knew the hurtful, and often brutal, way my grandmother had imposed her will on my mother when she was a small child, a teenager and then in a less harsh way as an adult. I also knew of the sadness Mum had experienced, left back in Jamaica, where her mother chose to leave her (or abandon depending on your perspective) at three years old. Albeit that she left her in the care of relatives which was the acceptable mode of the day with many Caribbean families. My grandmother was distant and cold and never connected with my mother, and this hurt me

Bigger Than the Moon

immensely. I was always on the offensive in her presence, determined to battle for the love that I felt my mother yearned for and deserved. I remember looking at her dying in the bed with its crisp white clinical sheets, and knew it was too late to understand why it was this way between them.

I stopped remembering as my thoughts were starkly interrupted by the sound of a horn announcing the docking of the ferry that had made its way over from the island. My right cheek felt damp as the wind gently blew against it, and I realised a tear had fallen quietly down my face. I moved my hand to wipe away the evidence of my sadness. Looking up, I saw that people had made their way off the ferry onto the pier. It was a small piece of decking that connected the boats docked to the dry land. I made a mental note to go and visit the island before I left to go back home. I am getting married this year and realise that my grandmother will not be alive to see it.

Generational cycles are negative patterns or traits. They are passed down from our family's history to several generations until someone decided to break these vicious cycles... Generational cycles can only be broken if we become fully aware of them...

— CONNECTIONS PARADISE BLOG —
WWW.CONNECTIONSPARADISE.COM

How will you know your guru? The guru will know you. You don't have to look for the guru. The guru appears when you are ready. You'll know... Even your enemies can be teachers who wake you up to a place that you're not... everyone and everything in the universe becomes your teacher and a means of awakening.

— RAM DASS, *POLISHING THE MIRROR*

Falling Apart

Autumn had always been my favourite season of the year. I love the 'crisp' air feeling that comes with its arrival and the refreshing winds that gently, or sometimes quite aggressively, spur on the inevitable separation of leaves from branches. The process of falling apart initiates the leaves' journey to the ground in order to renew and revitalise for the next season of growth. Autumn took on a different meaning once Chloe was born as it heralded the beginning of a particularly challenging time in my life. As 2009 commenced it did feel like one big loss and separation: a loss of my dreams and the reality I had intently built for myself and the crashing down of everything I thought was going to make me happy. It was, as one of my ex-bosses would sometimes say when coaching me through work issues, a 'teaching moment'. In fact, there were several teaching moments that were going to happen for me moving forward, but at this point I could not quite see where it was all leading me to. Chloe's birth and all the challenges that had come with it were still

Falling Apart

fresh, and present. I remained in a lot of pain physically, requiring regular visits to physical therapists to help me get better mobility. I was also dealing with Chloe's various health conditions that seemed to be getting worse. After the visit to the clinic for Chloe's heart, her dermatologist and GP agreed that given all the issues that had arisen, as well as the growing concerns that Chloe was not meeting her developmental milestones, she should be referred to a paediatrician. In February 2009 she attended an appointment to see Dr Collins. My health insurance continued to be a valuable support and the referral was pretty quick. Dr Collins physically examined Chloe. It was always painful for me to watch Chloe be tugged and pulled in physical exams (this had been one of many by this point). She was approaching five months old but in terms of all the experiences we had been through by this point, it felt like she was older. Chloe was still quite sore from the eczema and Dr Collins agreed with me that she was extremely hyper-mobile – her joints were flexible beyond the normal range and very 'loose'. She did not appear to demonstrate signs of holding her body up on her own, even slightly. She always needed some form of support, be that your hand or a pillow. I had also begun to notice a pattern of her rocking in her baby bouncer quite aggressively. It was like a set rhythm and increased with intensity when she heard music. This may not have seemed unusual to anyone else, and logically could have looked like a response to the music, a form of dancing even, but with my intuition on high alert it felt like something was going on; she always looked so intense and focused at the same time and I felt uncomfortable with what I observed. If I did mention my concerns to others, I would get the inevitable 'she's fine' in response and a sense that I was overthinking. Eventually, once Chloe was diagnosed, I realised this was 'stimming', a coping or self-soothing mechanism, but for now I made a note of everything to discuss with the medical professionals. I relayed my concerns to Dr Collins and, given his own observations, he said that she should be referred to the NHS consultant paediatrician team to be observed for a potential global developmental delay assessment.

I am forever grateful for the many professionals like Dr Collins who listened to me in those early days. Without them I don't know what would have happened to Chloe. There were many lessons I personally had to learn in the experience with Chloe, and one of the most important would be the art of listening; truly listening to yourself and others. You only really understand the art of listening and how important it is when you need to be heard! You realise what it takes and how hard it can be. Up until

Falling Apart

Chloe's birth I was not a great listener. I thought I was because I 'heard' everything and learnt at a very rapid pace. However, I was learning through this journey that listening is not about the speed and pace of receiving information. It is actually the opposite; it is about being present and patient and slowing down your own thought process so you can hear someone else's first and digest it, fully. Being heard during this time was a gift. One that would lead me to many sources and places of support, advice and help. By osmosis I also tried to do the same with people around me, knowing how much I had appreciated being listened to in the journey to understand what was happening with Chloe.

During this time I was also battling many personal challenges. I had to manage all the complexities of Chloe's development delay with the thought of going back to work, which was scheduled for the next couple of months. I put myself under such pressure; I felt uneasy with my return to work as my still very fragile body was taking a long time to recover. We also had to keep the world going for our son. I had started to go down the dark rabbit hole of comparing my daughter's growth and development to everyone else around her age. For the first time in my life I was confused, without a clue where to turn, who to confide in and how to move forward.

Bigger Than the Moon

I returned to work on a phased basis when Chloe was six months in April 2009. I realigned to a new role, with a fantastic leader to work for and a very challenging agenda for my first few months back. It was a very hard time for me, and many of my colleagues had no idea what I was going through, especially with Chloe. Should I have asked for more help and support at the time? Absolutely. Did I? No. Now I think women feel more empowered to ask for the support they need as the workplace is generally more evolved. Although I accept that this is not the case everywhere, even today.

My suggestion to anyone who is in the world of pre-diagnosis or in any time of immense change, whatever the situation, is to really embrace vulnerability. Be clear and honest with yourself first about what you need so that you can try to get the support that may be required. Being strong may require you to be weak for a while as you try to adjust to what is happening. Unfortunately at the time, I was almost soldier-like in my return to work in spite of the many challenging circumstances that I needed to navigate. I made myself look capable, confident and ready to go. On the plus side, I showed myself what I was capable of. I felt the need to keep up appearances and ensure everything stayed on track with my career. I put myself through what I can only describe as the mental equivalent of a marathon

Falling Apart

– without any of the preparation or training! I realise now that it was complete insanity and that what had been a strength of mine, to be able to do so much, was now becoming a weakness. At the time, however, it felt like I had no choice. Or maybe the truth was that it worked to serve as a distraction from what was happening to me in my personal life. Either way, I wanted so much for everything to be 'right' and 'normal'. I now know those two terms don't always co-exist in the reality of life. But that was then, and I was not yet ready to understand all of this. I wasn't yet fully awake.

To try to ease into working life – and on reflection in some way to continue my efforts to make everything 'right' – I had arranged a family holiday to Tobago in April 2009 to visit my friend who lived on the island with her family. Chloe's skin was still quite sore, but her eczema had become more controlled and I felt like the break would do us all good, giving us time to connect as a family of four, as well as benefitting from the therapy of sunshine and a different climate. I still hoped against hope that I could restore my dream of the life I had wanted and not the one it appeared I was transitioning to. I was still refusing to 'open the door' and stayed a little while longer in the room of denial. It was the first time Chloe had travelled and she was a dream baby as we went through

Bigger Than the Moon

the different stages of airport, airplane and landing. Che had also been a good traveller and his first trip abroad was at six months too. The experience I had travelling with my parents from a very young age made me realise that seeing the world was such a gift and offered invaluable educational opportunities for children that a classroom could not compensate for.

The holiday, however, merely served to illuminate the increasing gulf between myself and my children's father. We did share some lovely moments with our children on the trip, touring the island and being with friends. I remember taking a 'selfie' of the four of us on one of the most beautiful beaches on the island – Englishman's Bay. It was probably the last time that I would take a picture like that. What did continue, however, was the happy smiling faces of our children in that picture; whatever was to happen next in our respective journeys we would remain committed to their happiness and stability.

My return to work required that we start the dreaded search for the right childcare for Chloe. We initially identified a nursery for her that was near the house and had a fairly good reputation. It felt so hard to make the right choice for her and much harder than when we first put Che in a nursery at the same age. I had this silent unspoken sense of dread as I was conscious that Chloe's

Falling Apart

developmental milestones were delayed. She was still not sitting up on her own without support and needed a lot more care and attention physically. Chloe seemed so vulnerable and I therefore felt immense guilt. It also did not help that she was such a sweet-natured baby, and the thought of leaving her with strangers made this an even harder decision. There was no choice at the time: I had to go back to work as we could not afford another six months of me being off, being the primary breadwinner.

We also decided to go for an alternative approach given my concerns on Chloe's development and we hired a childminder so that Chloe's week was effectively split between nursery and childminder. The childminder was a referral, so in that sense I felt much more comfortable. Chloe's dad and I both liked her and she seemed to have a warm nature and took to Chloe quite well when we visited her home. Chloe also seemed relaxed with her and that was enough for me. It was settled then that Chloe would do three days at the childminder and two days at the nursery. I thought that being at the nursery would help with her development and allow her to be around other children thereby giving her more 'stimulation'.

At this point, however, everything started to unravel. In May 2009, Chloe caught chicken pox from the nursery, which I was initially extremely pleased about given my ultra-efficient approach to life, always wanting to be ahead of challenges. Chloe catching this at such an early age meant that it could just be over and done with. Her brother had caught it just after his first birthday, so I felt that this was one milestone I had managed to meet in front of time!

Chloe was still under observation with her consultant dermatologist for her eczema, which was a good thing as the chicken pox developed into something much worse. My return to work was staggered, so I was able to work part-time for the first month, which meant I could stay at home with Chloe as her chicken pox got progressively worse. One day the spots began to deteriorate into open sores. I could only imagine how she was feeling although she never cried and was silently accommodating this affliction that was getting worse by the day. I felt desperate, and I put a blanket over the top of the buggy so no one would see her as I made my way to the doctor's – her sores were red raw all over her face and now her body, some oozing pus from infection and others a darker red where they had started to become scabs.

The doctor saw her immediately when the staff in reception alerted him to her condition and what she looked like. As she was already under observation he said that I should take her to the consultant dermatologist straight

Falling Apart

away – Dr Manning fitted us in and so I bundled her up in her car seat and took her to the hospital outpatient department that had now become very familiar to her.

I remember Dr Manning's face was calm but shocked – she immediately phoned the A&E department to get Chloe assessed on an emergency basis as soon as possible. The look on her face was all I needed to see to know that this was a serious situation. We left the hospital with our son in tow (who we had managed to pick up from school in the middle of all of this) and took the drive down to the A&E department so that we could be seen by the consultant specialists. I lifted the car seat out of the car and carried it rather than attach it to the buggy, with Chloe safely tucked in and a blanket over the handle so no one could see her. My head was in a number of places at once: here with Chloe worrying about how serious her condition was, looking at Che thinking about how hungry he must be and that I would need to get him up for school the next morning, and then worrying about the meeting I needed to attend first thing, knowing how tired I would be. My head was swirling with all of these thoughts – but not for long as we made our way to the children's department and asked for the consultants. They quickly came down to meet us. One look at Chloe and they rushed us to an examination room.

Bigger Than the Moon

What followed was a horrendous couple of hours as Chloe was examined by the consultants from top to toe, and given how close the sores were around her eyes they informed us that the retinas and corneas of both her eyes would need to be examined to ensure the chicken pox had not attacked those areas. The process involved a clamp-like structure that allowed the doctors to examine the back of the eyes and they warned us it could be quite distressing to watch. I could not bear it and so Chloe's dad picked up the mantle and accompanied her with the doctors to the room where she would undergo the eye examination. He was always better in these situations, and I never functioned very well in a hospital environment at the best of times. I sat outside waiting with our son. It had been an exhausting day and evening. As the time went on, I remember sitting in the waiting room in a trance-like state, almost sleepy. It had been a hot sticky day in May and running around in the heat had also got to me. I was at a loss to understand what was happening. I would ask the question 'why?' many times over the next few years knowing that an answer very rarely arrived.

After this episode, Chloe undertook an intensive skin-care routine, overseen by Dr Manning, our now favourite person.

Metamorphosis

Summer 2009 saw Chloe's skin start to slowly recover, thanks to Dr Manning and her care and attention. It was as if the episode with her chicken pox was a crescendo of sorts in terms of the many issues that she had been battling with regarding her skin. I felt that this condition was a symptom of something much deeper that was trying to come out. I know it may sound very 'new-age' and not grounded in fact, but I was learning to lean into my intuition in a very unconscious way at this stage (it became more conscious over the next few years as I realised how powerful it was to listen more internally than externally). Chloe had now moved into a routine regarding the management of her physical challenges. She was still not able to lift herself up or crawl independently, and although she had started to get stronger sitting up on her own, she still required some support and was quite 'wobbly'.

Chloe was now approaching nine months old. It was a very physical job being her parent as you had to help

Bigger Than the Moon

her navigate any physical movement. I lifted Chloe everywhere! For me it was like she had a disability even before it was diagnosed; she needed an incredible amount of continuing help and supervision. I also had Che to think about, even though he was a dream older sibling. He would be my other set of ears and eyes if I could not have Chloe directly in my gaze for whatever reason. He instinctively knew he had a role with her and just naturally fell into it. I hope as he reads this he recognises what a special role he has played in Chloe's life, and I do feel that she was able to end up making the progress she did (and still does) in great part due to his constant presence in her life and the attention he gave her. He brought himself into her world and she in turn responded to this. Che is my hero, and I would turn to him often over those early years (and later) as we worked together with Chloe to ensure she was engaged, even if her behaviour suggested a desire to disconnect from engagement. She was very happy in her own company as a baby and fixated on things that did not require her to interact with anyone else. Che would always be able to find some way to engage with her. It was beautiful to see and this connection remains to this day.

At this stage Chloe was not communicating, even non-verbally, at a level that would be expected for her age, and this concerned me the most (next to her incessant rocking in her baby bouncer). I never knew if she was in pain or hurt, even during the severe chicken pox episode. Chloe only appeared very lethargic but never got 'upset' and didn't have the normal signals a baby would have in distress. I could only sense from the way she would look at me with her eyes. She was babbling and had started to appear to want to say 'Mumma' and 'Dadda', but it always felt like she was unsure. To me it seemed that nobody was that concerned apart from me and to a lesser extent her dad, who in this early stage was still more relaxed about the rate of her progress although he did observe there was a difference with Chloe. I had started to get frustrated that our closest relatives wanted to rationalise away my concerns, often citing my need for perfection to be the real issue and that Chloe was developing as she needed to. I guess at its core their perception was valid – but I refused to accept that her progress was 'normal'; I believed Chloe needed help and I was determined to make sure that happened, in spite of the way that some members of both our families waved away my concerns. The summer proceeded with Chloe eventually transitioning to her childminder full-time. I had returned to work full-time, and for me this was a chance to be in a mode that I was much more at ease with, and I felt I could be more in control in that space of work, doing what I

Bigger Than the Moon

was good at. This in turn increased my confidence and I think helped me start to rebuild my mental strength. I was always going to be a working mum, and for the first time I started to really embrace the idea and was building an inner pride around that. Chloe's childminder also looked after another girl who was a little bit younger than Chloe so there was the opportunity for some interaction. I knew the nursery was not the right place for her. I would pick Chloe up after a long day at work and equally long commute and arrive in the play room to see her lying on her back, slightly elevated with a pillow, under a baby arch with lots of toys on it, which she enjoyed. However, I could not help feeling that as she was not very responsive like other kids at this age, it was easy for nursery staff (often young and inexperienced) to leave her and not feel the need to stimulate her much or provide the right level of attention. I used to feel sad when I picked her up as she seemed not to be with other children. When I arrived to pick her up, however, she would always greet me with the biggest smile. My heart hurt for the amount of love I had for this delicate baby, and I always felt conflicted. I knew that she needed more help but having to combine supporting her with working full-time was something I battled with in those early years. I knew deep down that I was doing my best, but it was a feeling I could not shake.

Metamorphosis

Moving her to the childminder full-time intuitively felt like the right decision. I wanted her to be in a 'home' environment if she was going to be away from me for most of the day. The childminder's friendly family and her warm nature seemed to align with that. Chloe's dad and I would alternate pickups and drop-offs between us, which were managed around both our full-time working schedules. Che's school schedule was also becoming increasingly busy and reflective of an active six-year-old boy who was very much into every extra-curricular activity you could imagine.

For a while our world was centred around play-dates, PTA meetings, hospital/doctor appointments for Chloe, managing work schedules and visits to various family members at the weekend. Chloe had a further appointment with her heart consultant Dr Davis in June 2009. His letter to Chloe's GP was factual and suggested progress in the closing of the hole in her heart:

> I reviewed Chloe who is now eight months of age. She is very well and there are no concerns. On examination, she was well and pink and all her peripheral pulses were present including her femorals. She had normal cardiac impulses with a normal first and second heart sound with a short

> systolic murmur 1/6, which was loudest at the lower left sternal edge... In conclusion, I am pleased to report that as Chloe is growing the VSD is reducing in size and now has some tissue within it in addition. I am sure that this will close in the short to midterm and is highly unlikely to ever require intervention. She needs no especial precautions and I would like to see her again in four months...

It seemed poignant that as Chloe's heart was starting to close, I needed to open mine to a new reality. It was around Chloe's first birthday in October 2009 that I started to become much more aware of the emotional door that I needed to open and walk through. Up until this point I had been on a sort of personal automatic pilot. Whilst I was fully aware and functioning both as a parent focused on Chloe's and Che's needs as well as working in a busy corporate environment, I had put my personal issues and my sense of emotional and physical well-being to the side.

Chloe's first birthday marked the beginning of me sensing a shift. I had started to realise that I was going to need to be stronger than I currently was to manage what I believed was going to be a long journey for Chloe and for me. During this time, I felt as if I was looking at things from the outside; similar to the feeling I had when I was

Metamorphosis

giving birth to her. We had decided to have a family birthday party for Chloe, which would mean the house being mostly flooded with Chloe's dad's side of the family (he has such a big family!) and just a few of mine and some of our mutual friends. It felt unusual to me because it was such a familiar scene but I had begun to feel different. Everyone was acting as if things were normal, but they were not.

I remember the scene. It was the usual noise of a birthday party for a one-year-old. Cousins of all ages were running around and aunts and uncles talking in a symphony all at once but each making sense in their own conversations. Food was in abundance, very typical of a Caribbean family get-together, and music accompanied the sounds and smells. The house was rich with family and laughter. A relative was sitting with Chloe at the dining table, holding her as she sat her small frame on the tabletop. Chloe still could not sit up on her own very strongly. She was flopping almost unstable in the relative's hands. As I noted the lack of steadiness, pointing it out and looking, in fact, almost yearning, for someone to share my observations and fears, the relative clinically dismissed my concerns (in a tone of frustration that I think was more about an irritation with me than my concerns) with words to the effect that Chloe was 'fine'.

Bigger Than the Moon

I knew then that Chloe was not fine. It was this strong sense of intuition but now it was becoming validated by clear observations. Chloe continued to stare intensely almost with a focus beyond that of the natural curiosity of a one-year-old. Although not entirely disconnected from her environment she seemed to be observing it from a different place. I had also noticed that she needed to be prompted for affection. She would not naturally reach out for you or react emotionally to situations. In spite of this her dad, brother and I showered her with love and kisses, even if we did not get that much back in return. We loved beyond limits, and I do believe that this was important in later developments with Chloe. The one thing Chloe did do was smile sometimes to herself, perhaps having seen something in her environment we may not have noticed or when observing her mad brother who at this age was a typical boisterous six-year-old rolling, tumbling, jumping and kicking a football all over the house. Chloe's birthday came and went but my feeling of unease remained.

During this time I also started to suffer from a pain in my inner ear. I embarked on numerous visits to specialists who performed a multitude of tests that found a perfectly functioning inner and outer ear with no issues either in my ears, or connected areas of my nose and throat. It was awful and started to affect my ability to sleep, and I

Metamorphosis

even started to lose my balance with episodes of dizziness. Looking back this was all probably physical symptoms of stress (and mild vertigo) but my sense of personal well-being was practically non-existent at this point. I was so focused on Chloe and also parenting Che who needed me just as much for different reasons. There seemed to be no time to stop. It was relentless and there was also a lot happening at work. I didn't realise then that the issues I was facing were my body's way of telling me to stop. I ended up being diagnosed with an inner ear imbalance due to a viral infection that required vestibular physiotherapy. My world was indeed spinning around me.

A couple of months after Chloe's first birthday, we decided to take a family trip to Florida. It was December 2009; my sister was going to join us, and we would be there through to the New Year. It was such a great time being with my sister, who adored her niece and nephew and who also helped to neutralise the unspoken distance that was increasing between myself and their dad. All of us had some beautiful moments on this holiday and although it would never be the same again, I knew the memories would be important.

It was during this holiday that I got to focus on the things I had been observing in Chloe and her development but see it in a different setting. I knew I was going to need to make some changes and take action once we returned home. It was fascinating watching Chloe that first night when we arrived at the resort. I still have the picture to this day of her sitting on the bed – with a soft support cushion – staring in wonderment and, it also seemed, with a little fear, at the spinning of the overhead ceiling fan. She just stared constantly at it, like it was making so much more noise and sensation than the rest of us could understand or comprehend. I remember looking at her with a reassuring face, so that she knew it was okay, and telling her what it was, but she only looked at me momentarily before switching her fixed gaze back towards the ceiling, still looking overwhelmed by this whizzing, spinning giant above her head.

There was time on this holiday to be still, with no distraction of the normal day-to-day routine of my life at home with work and caring for Chloe and Che. I would come to learn the importance of taking moments to stop and be in silence which would eventually be something I applied in my life as a result of this journey with Chloe. I had the chance to be with her totally and 'see' and acknowledge what I had been sensing for a while. She was both connecting with us but also disconnecting quite clearly into her own world. We would visit the theme parks and she would smile with the characters when prompted by

Metamorphosis

us, but there were moments when she appeared to just be in her own world focusing intently on something or just looking serious observing a ride. I remember a picture I took with her as I lay on a lounger by the pool one day and she was lying across my leg. Her face is at the centre of the photo, and she is deep in thought looking out into the distance somewhere, holding my leg with her tiny hands, so that I could know she was also with me. That picture remains one of my favourites of Chloe and me, as it was the one that accurately conveyed the moment that I started to move into a new reality. It was one that was scary for me, but I knew was necessary. I had to open the door and find a way to help her, and in some way I also had to find out how to help myself.

Abre la puerta! Open the door!

— DR CLARISSA PINKOLA ESTES

Midway along the journey of our life
I woke to find myself in a dark wood,
for I had wandered off from the straight path.

— DANTE, *INFERNO*

The Middle

This part of the journey is hard to reflect on. I was managing a lot of things all at once at this time, which was, in many ways, an extremely traumatic experience for me. In the process of recalling and remembering, I was instantly taken back to all the surrounding events and subsequent emotions that I went through.

The middle in most stories of personal challenge is a hard place but it is where the process of transformation really happens, as well as the learning. I often say when managing and coaching individuals I work with in times of change and disruption that the process of 'changing' never feels good. When you do eventually arrive at the destination or outcome, you will remember these moments and see them as times that built your fortitude, strength and resilience. It's important to note, however, that this may not be true for all situations. I want to be clear that sometimes people don't and just can't make it, for whatever reason. I believe it is important to acknowledge that: everyone's journey is different, and life can be hard, unkind and unbearable for many people for many different reasons. There are so many things you need within and outside of you to support the journey and sometimes even that may not be enough for some people.

For me, there were moments in the following few years which were truly hard. I became even more isolated at home and then at work as I was trying to balance keeping everything together and deliver to my normal high standards. As a mother at the school gates with the other parents who appeared ('appeared' is used deliberately as more often than not they were battling challenges just as much as me) to be living idyllic happy lives. Many of the parents were stay-at-home, but not all. Much of the focus for many of them was worrying about PTA issues and how to prepare their children for the inevitable private / selective secondary schools which they were all battling to ensure entry into. Long-ago feelings from my childhood were starting to appear, but in a different way. The school gates were like the playground setting of my childhood where I never felt as if I belonged; a bit of a 'No Man's Land'. Being everywhere (I worked full-time and also joined the PTA) and belonging nowhere. Chloe was different from other children her age. I had always felt different, and I began to identify at a very deep emotional level with what I knew she was going to go through because of this.

The Middle

I recall being sensitive to any notion or observation on Chloe's development. This came from everywhere and very well intended, casual comments: 'Is she walking yet?' 'Any words yet?' 'She is sooo good – doesn't make any trouble' rang in my head like the sound of drums as I smiled through it all, explaining away that she was 'taking her time'. I probably put more pressure on myself, but it made me realise how people don't often take the time to just pause and think that everyone has a story or something they are going through and if only we stayed a bit more in the space of silence, we may realise that. I started to recede from my life into an internal mental space where only I was present and knew how I really felt.

I had opened the door and stepped into an unknown space to me. It began in February 2010 when Chloe was referred to a consultant community paediatrician, Dr Oliver. After returning from that holiday in January 2010, I was resolved to actively pursue some sort of outcome or diagnosis for Chloe. Nobody was calling it autism at that point. I did not know what it was, but I knew it was something. What was also clear was that inaction was not going to get us anywhere and more importantly provide the support Chloe needed. Was I thinking about her 'getting better' at this stage? In some sense, probably yes. In my mind it was a case of finding out what was wrong

Bigger Than the Moon

and then 'fixing it'. I was so desperate to 'fix it' like most things in my life where things were not going as planned. I was not yet ready to accept at this point, but it was still early and more needed to happen for this realisation to take place. I had to push and force the inquiry into Chloe's development delay and bring a voice to the concerns that were now becoming overwhelming for me.

Equally, at work it was the end of a very intense period in the agenda I had been asked to take the lead on after returning from maternity leave. I was working for an amazing leader who was a wonderful person and full of humour, compassion and integrity. I respected him and I believe he respected me and the work I did. He understood that I was coming to a point in my career where I wanted to do something different. I had been with the same company, straight from university, for twelve years at this stage and it felt like I was shifting into a new phase in my life in more ways than one. My experience as a HR professional came in handy at this stage. I knew it was important to ready myself for this next phase – but I was not sure what the next phase was. However, it was important to take action in order to trigger momentum, wherever that was leading me. I am still in touch with this individual, who, even now, I know I can count on to find time for me. This was the first point I realised the power

The Middle

of the network; the importance of surrounding yourself with a support system which was to become a critical part of my journey and experience both on a personal and professional level.

While pondering what was next, I was head-hunted for a very different kind of opportunity in the world of financial services. It was just two years after the 2008 crisis and possibly the worst (or best depending on your perspective) time to join the world of banking and that was exactly what appealed to me (in my insane need for stretch and challenge). My world was becoming disrupted in every way and it felt like this opportunity fitted into how I wanted to feel during this time; anonymous. I had grown up in my first company, got married and now had two children. Colleagues had started to become firm friends and knew everything about me. My personal life was about to be disrupted and I felt that it would be liberating to go through that in a place where nobody really knew me and where I didn't have to explain anything; it felt like a blank canvas and well timed. I yearned to have some part of my life where I was anonymous and could effectively 'start again'. It goes without saying the role was a fantastic opportunity too; I was asked to reengineer the recruitment agenda across the Europe Middle East and Africa (EMEA) region and build a centre of excellence

Bigger Than the Moon

model across the 52 countries that this region covered. It felt like the kind of challenge where I knew I could make an impact and it was different. I had built my business career as a HR generalist in the main and this was an opportunity to specialise in an area of expertise in a totally different industry. Talent acquisition, or recruitment as it was then commonly known, was starting to become an area of increasing focus for businesses at that point, especially with the emerging technology landscape. I saw the potential to develop my skills and expertise in something that I knew would become a critical capability for business (and I was proved right with, of course, some helpful guidance and counsel from people in my network at the time).

I also loved the idea of going somewhere and being the new person with everything to prove: the long-acquired habit from childhood of proving myself was something I would eventually get over as my career developed. It proved in many ways to be the thing I had to master in both my professional and personal life.

Quotes noted in my journal at various points in 2010

> Cows run away from the storm while the buffalo charges toward it – and gets through it quicker. Whenever I am confronted with a tough challenge, I do not prolong the torment, I become the buffalo.
>
> – WILMA MANKILLER, THE FIRST FEMALE PRINCIPAL CHIEF OF THE CHEROKEE

> For I know the plan I have for you, says the Lord. You will seek me and find me; when you seek me with all your heart I will be found by you, says the Lord.
>
> – JEREMIAH 29:11

Buffalo

The year 2010 was the year I learned to lean in to my intuition in an active way. I had begun to journal with a clear objective and focus. I had always noted life events and musings in the form of writings of various sorts, but this was different. It felt very intentional. I am not sure what started the process but I realised I needed some way to externalise the inner reflections I had. This more focused attempt to journal was, I guess, my way of preparing myself for the road ahead. It acted as a prompt, a guide, inspiration and in some ways I used it as a way of building my strength and sharpening my focus for what I knew I was going to have to manage and go through. I did not have any real clarity on what lay ahead for me. There was just a sense that it was going to be tough, long and would require a resilience to manage what was, quite frankly, unprecedented territory for me.

I was going to head into the storm straight on. No left turn or shortcut. I was ready to do the work and dig deep. I had started to collect clippings from magazines and quotes from books and had created a vision board process in the journal itself as well as writing. The clippings were mainly from lifestyle magazines and anything with travelling as a theme. There were images of the ocean, solitary figures lying on a beach, places I wanted to visit and most of all images that conveyed how I wanted to feel when this was all over. It was like visual intention setting and it focused me. I wrote anything that came into my mind; how I was feeling, working through the thoughts and fears of the transition I was undertaking, both in work and my personal life – the decisions I needed to make and the changes I needed to create. I was definitely very scared and knew my world, as I currently experienced it, was about to change for good. I also clung tightly to that long-held belief given to me by my wonderful parents; 'nothing good comes easy'. I knew that something better was going to be waiting for me if I just stepped into this scary place of uncertainty. Whilst it was Chloe's condition that triggered the work, I realised that it was a process that was entirely about me. I knew I could not help Chloe if I did not look at the work I needed to do with myself and the situation I had found myself in at this point in my life. It was taking me away from myself and who I was; I needed to find myself again and also in some ways become who I was destined to be in order to be in the best possible position to help Chloe. What was hard in those early days pre-diagnosis was having to do that work in parallel and keep the world turning for my son Che as well. It took all my strength to keep going. In all of this I looked like the swan effortlessly working hard at my job, caring for my children, and in many ways keeping up a pretence of normality so as not to alert people too quickly to this process of awakening that I was going through; I needed to prepare first.

At the beginning of 2010 through to the summer, Chloe was continuing her medical journey. Her medical letters in February 2010 note the numerous investigative tests that her consultant paediatrician had sent her for as part of the elimination process of what Chloe potentially could have: haemoglobin and full blood count, thyroid function tests, urea and electrolytes, serum creatine kinase, plasma amino acids, chromosome analysis and search for Fragile X. She had also prescribed urine tests: urinary amino acids, urinary organic acids. The chromosome test required her to be sedated so that she could be put through a MRI scanner. She was only fifteen months at this point and her dad and I watched with a sense of fear and amusement as, a few minutes after taking the medicine, she gradually stumbled into unconsciousness when the sedative took hold. We quickly caught her before she reached the ground.

Buffalo

Chloe could not walk well, or strongly, unaided at this point and was still very vulnerable and it took a lot of strength from both of us to watch her go through all these tests – however, I knew they were necessary and I was grateful for Dr Oliver's attention to my daughter's development issues. I needed to know that someone else other than her dad and I were looking out for her to understand what was going on. Advocacy for your child must also come from other sources and not just yourself; whilst you are the best one, you need others to join you in order to get the best support for your child – it's critical to be relentless in seeking out your co-advocates. Her dad had now also fully aligned with my concerns around Chloe's development and this was helpful for me as it meant I no longer felt like a lone voice and it strengthened our ability to collectively work together in order to get an outcome for Chloe determined.

Dr Oliver had noted, following an assessment of Chloe to her GP, that:

> Parents say she is not walking independently but is now beginning to pull herself up to stand. She can be left sitting on the floor for long periods and crawls symmetrically. She is also quite sociable, laughs loudly during turn-taking games and keeps

well to her daily routine. Her hearing and vision are normal... Chloe walks with a slightly wide base gait when led by both her hands. She has quite hyper-extensible joints at the knees and her ankles. Her development was assessed using the Griffiths Mental Development Scales... Chloe engaged well in the assessment... she shouts for attention, made some reciprocal babble with a string of vowel sounds... she is just beginning to attempt brick building... Overall Chloe's development is within the lower average range for her age...

Dr Oliver went on to say that the agreed plan for Chloe was as follows: 'referral to physiotherapy, referral to Early Years and Portage team for input.' She also noted: 'parents to consider registering Chloe to attend any of the Early Years Centres close to the family home.'

She also organised for Chloe to have a chromosomal karyotype because of her VSD and the fact that I had polyhydramnios during my pregnancy. As Chloe was at her childminder full-time, visits by the Portage team would take place in the childminder's home with her dad mostly in attendance as he was able to be more flexible to make appointments during the day than I was. My passion and commitment for flexible working really

Buffalo

grew during this period; I would not have been able to grow my career and keep the world turning for both my children if I had not experienced this flexibility and being able to continue to work. I am proud that I can continue the work promoting the benefits of this today as part of my professional role. So many parents of children with special needs (and even children without any specific needs) have to give up work at this point and so begins the socio-economic divide as well as the impact on many parents, affecting mostly women, having to put aside their own needs and capabilities in order to have to make choices between their children and their personal aspirations and dreams. Whilst this is an intensely personal choice, I think it is important that parents do have that genuine choice and if they so choose, can be supported in continuing their professional lives whilst also continuing to support their children's needs. In my view this is important for society as a whole and in the effort to be truly inclusive.

In April 2010, we had a follow-up appointment for Chloe with Dr Davis to assess progress with her VSD. Chloe was eighteen months at this point. His assessment was that she had a normal cardiovascular examination and that he was unable to hear a murmur but that she was not very still. In conclusion his letter to our local GP states that,

I'm pleased to report that as Chloe is growing, the VSD is reducing in size. I am still hoping that this will close in the short to the mid-term, but even if it does not it is highly unlikely to ever require intervention. I would like to see her again in six months, and she needs no especial precautions.

A month later in May 2010 her cytogenetics report noted that 'The presence of the fragile X chromosome was excluded at the 3% level with 95% confidence and a normal female karyotype.'

We followed up with Dr Oliver for another assessment at the end of May. Her report following this assessment to our local GP noted that Chloe was now nineteen months old. This assessment was for me another validation of my sense that something more was going on with Chloe and that her developmental delay was more than just that. However, at this point Dr Oliver was careful not to draw early conclusions:

I saw Chloe for a review of her progress… She is now one year and seven months old. She attended with her parents who report progress in all areas of Chloe's development… She is now crawling, pulls to

Buffalo

stand and side-steps around furniture. Her hand skills have also improved. She enjoys looking at books and playing with musical cause and effect toys. She is also reported to be sociable and has a good understanding of her daily routine. She has one recognisable word and may recite children's rhymes. Chloe tends to moan to make requests and may rock herself to and fro. She calls to her mother by name (mum) only when she has to, however she is reported to be chatty to her brother whom she likes to observe while he is playing games or dancing. She gets quite excited and may clap her hands, rocks or hand-shakes during these times. At her childminder's, Chloe is reported to be sociable with other children.

She was observed in clinic to play with varied toys, especially cars; she was quite content on her own. She also enjoys some container play and playing with the puzzle form boards on the Griffiths Mental Developmental Scales. She showed improvements overall and developmentally she is at 14–16 months but her speech is slightly delayed at 11–12 months. She made very good eye contact. Chloe is self-directed in play... She has good attention. From my discussion with parents, she has some odd patterns of play and behaviour, such as showing some motor mannerisms (rocking, hand-shaking, or clapping when excited, watching her own reflection and looking excessively at lights). These together with her speech delay raises questions about a mild social communication difficulty however Chloe is quite young now and needs to be monitored.

Her next review was noted for six months' time and the intent was to continue with the current therapy plan. Part of this was to undergo a speech and language therapy assessment. This took place in June and July 2010. In the meanwhile, at work I had not spoken too much of the challenges I was having with Chloe as I was not really clear yet what those challenges were, but I was fortunate to work with someone who just 'got it' and worked with me to help coach and guide my thinking. This type of support in your workplace is invaluable; it is truly gold dust. That summer I was able to balance the needs of my professional work with managing the myriad of appointments that Chloe had to attend, all the time working in partnership with her dad.

The summary of the Speech and Language report indicated that there were concerns noted for both attention and listening skills and play skills. The report went on to say:

Buffalo

In the assessment Chloe enjoyed cause-and-effect toys where she could press buttons. She threw some toys. She knocked down a tower. She put a spoon into a cup and on a plate but did not pretend to eat. She enjoyed playing a game where the Speech and Language therapist pretended to eat, but did not imitate. Chloe's parents reported she does not carry out pretend play at home, but she does imitate what they do with the remote control, she stands and points it at the TV. Her parents reported she enjoys exploratory play and physical chasing games. She has begun trying to place pieces in inset puzzles.

They noted further areas of concern with understanding of language and use of language and stated that they would continue 'to monitor' other areas such as speech sound skills and eating/drinking/oro-motor skills. The report noted the following:

> Chloe makes vowel and consonant sounds and some non-speech noises like squealing… Chloe's eating and drinking skills have been delayed but she has recently begun to chew and she can now feed herself… Chloe has a delay in her attention and listening, play, understanding and use of language

> related to her developmental delay. She seems keen to communicate and initiates communication with adults. Her oro-motor and speech sound development require monitoring as they develop.

These reports, together with my own observations of Chloe at home, proved there were very real differences between her and her peer group in various settings. This made it seem increasingly certain that she had a special need. I knew that there was a diagnosis of some sort pending.

The health professionals had started to prepare us for the word 'autism'. They had suggested that autism could be a potential condition but would need a formal assessment. We were told that a formal diagnosis could only happen when Chloe was a minimum of three years old. As I started to do my research I realised that it was not common in the UK at that time (unlike in the US) to diagnose this early, and the tendency was to wait until they reached school age. My gut was telling me that would be too late and Chloe could get lost in the system, and that surely to diagnose before starting school would ensure she ended up in the right place for her. I had no idea what I was dealing with, but it felt right to battle for the assessment at three years old. It helped that we had a very attentive medical professional in Dr Oliver who agreed that an assessment at three would, at the very least, be helpful in ensuring the right early intervention plan for Chloe. What followed for the next year were therapies, appointments and regular assessments of Chloe's progress.

During the autumn I finalised the decision to take up the offer of the new role and there began the next phase of my career for what I initially planned to be two years. I ended up staying there just over eleven years: you never know what is going to happen in life and the new company would turn out to be a place of support, growth and learning in what was going to be a very tumultuous and eventful period of my life.

First Steps

Chloe's first stumbling steps were taken on New Year's Eve, December 2010. It felt poignant that as I was taking my first steps into this new scary place of discovery in work and life, she was venturing to do the same with her body and tiny feet. She and I were in her bedroom, and it was a special moment I will always remember. Chloe was 26 months old and was not able to walk independently at all up until this point. Her frame was very slim but she was tall and strong and it took a lot of strength to carry her: I had developed the upper body strength of a titan by this stage! We had to carry her everywhere and even little seven-year-old Che would attempt to lift her when she needed to go somewhere or reach something – it was so cute watching them.

Her signal to move would be to raise her arms as she was still not talking fluently and could not articulate her needs very well. On this particular evening, she and I sat on the floor in her bedroom and faced each other. She was doing her usual smiling at me and I looked at her; we

First Steps

both knew what was coming. I had been doing a routine with her where I would try and get her to take steps in her bedroom as she was settling for the evening and this was going to be another one of our attempts. I would encourage her to try to hold herself up and stand on her feet, albeit that I would take her soft delicate hands into mine to give her a sense of security. She would wobble and sway given the weakness of her gait area and her challenges with gross motor skills and reduced stability (as noted in her earlier medical assessment by Dr Oliver). I knew that she could do it, however, and this particular evening, I said to her in encouraging words, 'Come on, Chloe, you can do it! You can do it!' and suddenly contrary to our normal routine, I decided to let go of her hands. She looked at me, swerving from side to side but deciding to hold her hands out.

'This was it!' I said to myself. In order to let her believe, I had to show her that I believed she could do it, so I moved back and knelt on the floor about a metre away. She was laughing and smiling and wobbling all at the same time and I could see her digging deep. With a swift move of one foot she quickly followed with the other and then repeated the step twice before collapsing into my arms which she could see were waiting for her. This moment was to be repeated so many times for different milestones in Chloe's life. But this was the first step; the first moment she and I learned to partner to meet a goal. I felt hopeful.

I look back at this moment and realise that whilst I thought I was helping Chloe with this act of supporting her first steps, she was actually helping me; the power of letting go is immense and I learnt that letting go of Chloe and allowing her to know her own ability was a very important thing. This can be said for any child but for children with special needs you are extremely protective and ever watchful over them and it can be hard to let go because of your fears for what they may not be able to do, or what could happen to them. However, it is important at moments when you are both ready, to let go and face the fears head on.

I shouted for her brother who was next door in his bedroom and she repeated the act for him and then her dad came rushing up from downstairs – we were all laughing and hugging her and I had tears in my eyes. Chloe had achieved an important milestone and I knew from this moment that it reinforced what I had always felt, which was that I had to keep believing in her so that I could ensure others did too.

I had been at my new organisation a couple of months by this time and 2011 was a very busy first year in a role that was both demanding and exciting. Citi is one of

First Steps

the largest banks in the world and when I joined it was operating in over 160 countries. I felt like I had arrived in a huge organisation and struggled to understand how I was going to get my arms around it (which I of course eventually did). I feel very strongly about the role of HR in an organisation and its contribution to business performance. Working with so many people across my career to this point, I was fortunate to see some of the very best examples of leaders in this space. The journey I was going through with Chloe served to support my own personal development at work. I said earlier that I had become a better listener, and I realised the importance of having clear goals and purpose as I worked through the challenges with Chloe. In work I started to bring this learning in to the way I approached setting strategies and agendas and making sure the team were the most important part of the process (Oh, how I learnt the value of the team when it came to the medical and care professionals helping me with Chloe!). I also realised the importance of measurement of progress and always made sure in any work around the people agenda that the productivity was clear and that there was solid engagement for anything we were doing – and if not – a plan to get it. Chloe has been a great teacher for me personally as well as professionally.

Bigger Than the Moon

In Citi, I felt like I was able to take this approach to the next level, with so many people across the world to do some fantastic HR work with. There were major programmes of work that had to be delivered in my first year. I also had to build relationships with a new team which included getting them to trust me and believe in the vision of what I felt we could achieve. I was lucky to work with some very talented people.

Meanwhile on the personal front, I had also made the decision to separate from the children's dad. I knew I had to bring to a close the challenges I had been experiencing in this part of my personal life. I had to focus my energies on Chloe and Che, and by not addressing what else was going on in my personal life, I couldn't devote as much energy to them as I needed to. It was a very painful time. I had a few close friends who I confided in and only spoke to my line manager at work, the amazing Daryl, about what was happening. He knew that all I needed was the space to be able to deal with what was occurring in my life, so that I could continue to be effective at work. I am so grateful for the understanding and coaching he provided me, all without judgement. He just listened and was there when I needed guidance and support. How lucky I was to be surrounded by genuinely caring people who were human beings first and foremost. Life had landed me in

First Steps

the right place in order for me to be able to navigate this journey. Looking back it was a gift and I am grateful to the angels for guiding me. An important lesson: If you are working during these moments of transition, try to be brave and find people at work you can confide in, who can provide you with the space to be able to keep going. Vulnerability is key in the process of managing yourself in times of challenge – whatever that challenge is.

In the separation good and bad things happened. The good was that I realised who was in my corner in terms of friends and that I was able to continue to co-parent with their dad so that our children never felt a loss of love, just the loss of two parents no longer together. We showed up as a unit for anything to do with them: hospital appointments, school events/plays, helping out at school fayres, parents' evening, sport events and coordinating extra-curricular activities. I look back on my emails during this time and it was full of activity; I had become a school governor (with a short stint as a Chair) at a local primary school, managed to also get myself on my son's school's PTA and was working throughout. I think I was filling my life up with so many additional responsibilities as a way to cope with the many uncertain things that were happening around me. I don't think I was conscious of this at the time, and whilst it may sound slightly contrary, I

Bigger Than the Moon

believe it helped me to manage my life better and brought a sense of control to parts of my life. On reflection, I am both equally impressed and slightly overwhelmed at what I was able to do during those times. The ability to remain a parenting team was critical. Of course, it was not always easy and required me to rise above ego and feelings felt at the time but I knew it was important for my children's well-being and emotional development to do this. Later on as they grew older, this proved the right path for us to take. It's been very fulfilling, even if hard work, to raise two happy well-adjusted children together.

The bad was that overnight, literally, I lost a whole and significant part of my life. Most of my ex-husband's family never spoke to me once we separated: it was a silent separation with no noise. It would be eight whole years before I would be in contact with them again, and only due to him falling ill. I did not understand where this absence of caring came from, but I learned to accept it. It was painful to experience but I knew that something was guiding me to a better place with different people who would be for me. This story had come to an end with the door firmly shut behind me. I believed I was being pushed to move in a different direction and felt almost compelled to do so at this point; even though it was very hard and very slow work.

First Steps

It took a few months for us to work through the transition of physically separating but in September 2011 we established a co-parenting arrangement where the children stayed with him twice a week overnight and every other weekend. As life started again for me on my own I had no idea how I was going to make it work. I had become the buffalo and was ready now to go through the heart of the storm and focus on the process of getting a diagnosis for Chloe. I had cleared the decks of uncertainty and doubt: the clarity I was feeling was undeniable. I had made space in my life by making the decisions I had over the last three months and now could be laser focused on ensuring that Chloe could get the support she needed.

> Intuition is not to be consulted once and then forgotten. It is not disposable. It is to be consulted at all steps along the way, whether the woman's work be clashing with a demon in the interior, or completing a task in the outer world. It does not matter whether a woman's concerns and aspirations are personal or global. Before all else action begins with strengthening the spirit.
>
> — DR CLARISSA PINKOLA ESTES,
> *WOMEN WHO RUN WITH WOLVES*

Discovery

Prior to Chloe's formal assessment for autism and during the summer of 2011 we had decided to move Chloe from her childminder to a private nursery full-time. Her childminder had proved a great support during the past couple of years but I was starting to get concerned that Chloe was not getting the right level of peer interaction that I thought would help aid her development, especially on a social level. She had developed a habit where she would be right up at the television with her small hands stuck to the face of the TV, looking straight into the screen, mesmerised and stimulated by the light (later on this would be diagnosed as a form of sensory processing needs). I observed this on a few occasions when I picked her up and also sometimes at home.

We thought Chloe would benefit from the peer-to-peer stimulation provided by a nursery setting, still hoping that development delay, more than any specific special need, was the root cause of her issues. To support the transition, we initially sent her part-time to nursery

Bigger Than the Moon

and then full-time in the same year (September 2011). Chloe was now walking quite independently although she needed to wear some ankle-height 'Kickers' boots to help keep her stable and strengthen her gait as she walked, as recommended by the physiotherapists. She still had this tendency to sway and be quite stiff (which lasts to this day with a diagnosis in her teenage years of Development Coordination Disorder aka dyspraxia). We also noticed that she got tired quite easily. It clearly took a lot of effort for her to walk and be physical. At first, her time in the nursery was working out well and we expected the Portage teams to move their observation of Chloe from the childminder into the nursery setting. But something new had started to develop as she began to interact with other children: the dreaded meltdowns.

Meltdowns are one of the most significant and primary signs of autism, especially in younger children. It's also one of the reasons why there can be high instances of misdiagnosis or no diagnosis at all. These meltdowns are often confused with the seemingly normal actions of a 'terrible twos' toddler, although on closer examination they are different. So the challenge at Chloe's age was that it aligned, from a timing perspective, with the dreaded toddler tantrums which looked pretty similar. Che at the same age was a boisterous child with lots of

Discovery

energy and a formidable will, but there was always a limit to his tantrums and he would calm down much quicker. With Chloe it was different, almost as if you could not control it and neither could she. For a while I would go to pick up Chloe and these 'meltdowns' would be explained away as Chloe 'having a bad day'. The nursery team there for the most part loved her and there were a couple of people who she particularly gravitated towards and intuitively connected with. From a very early age, Chloe always seemed to have a highly tuned 'sixth sense' or 'intuition', which often played out in who she easily connected with, who she ignored and who she reacted to in certain situations (still does).

Interacting with other children was clearly becoming an issue for Chloe. It was, first of all, simple things like fixating on a specific toy or book and not being able to 'take turns'. She also continued to be very happy in her own company and playing solo, except of course when it came to her brother Che.

Some days I would pick her up and she had had 'a good day' but then the frequency of the 'bad days' started to increase. I was finishing long days at work, managing very complex agendas and stakeholders across the world, then going to pick up Chloe before rushing to pick up Che. There would always be this feeling of dread before I rang the nursery doorbell. They had typically contacted me beforehand at work, often during a meeting, to give me advance warning that Chloe was having a 'bad day' and the dread would start from then. Once I had arrived at the nursery, I would be greeted by the inevitable look of concern on the face of the nursery manager who would explain to me that 'Chloe's day had not been great.' What was more concerning to me was that nobody seemed to be able to say how they were going to help Chloe in the setting. I realised that it was going to be down to me to try to find a way forward so Chloe could get the support she needed.

I had done everything in my power to equip the nursery with the support from the local authority that Chloe had been receiving from the Portage team. I sent emails connecting them to the team directly, provided notes and guidance that we had been receiving and even arranged for the team to go and visit Chloe and staff in the actual setting. However, the nursery still seemed almost lazy and binary in their focus to outline the reasons why this was becoming an 'issue' for them. Equally, the local authority was refusing to attend to Chloe's needs in the nursery setting as the location was in another local authority area. So began the issues of cross-borough funding where neither local authority was willing to support, but clearly

Discovery

knew that one of them had to. The only person suffering during this time was Chloe. I wanted the nursery to be able to work with me to offer additional help and solutions and got met with very basic responses. The management team were clearly only focused on the issue from a financial resourcing perspective as Chloe clearly needed more help and attention in the setting from their staff, and they did not want to fund that. They also had other parents' complaints to manage as well, given the tantrums and disruption this would cause for other children, although I was less sympathetic about that.

This made it even more critical that her formal assessment for autism took place as soon as she reached her third birthday. My inner voice was speaking very loud and clear at this point. It also made me quite vocal about the lack of training, expertise and accountability in the private nursery industry when it came to matters like this and I felt they were lacking in their duty of care to Chloe.

The appointment for Chloe's autism assessment took place shortly after her third birthday. I was relieved it was finally happening but anxious about what it would conclude. I remember going into the room with her dad sitting next to me. It was still quite strained between us but at moments like that we remained a constant support for one another and each other's metaphorical shoulder

Bigger Than the Moon

to lean on when it came to anything to do with Chloe and Che. I was scared as, by then, I knew what the assessment was going to say.

I watched as Chloe sat at the little table and chair made especially for little people and she was asked to complete a series of tasks. Dr Oliver was present with another medical professional. I made a mental note of how they talked to her and engaged with her; they didn't rush the interaction. They were patient and present, watching her look at the books she was given. Eventually, after a bit of time passed, they got her to look through a book and asked her questions. First sign I observed: she kept flipping through the pages, not in a way that signalled a lack of interest but an almost obsessive repetition to go through each page and scan and then start again. She rebuffed attempts to ask questions about what she was reading and observing, sometimes answering with 'yes' and 'no' but mostly ignoring. Second sign I observed during the assessment: she wanted to line toys up – mainly cars. We had noted this at home, but I had not done too much research on autism as I was avoiding using any labels, so I had not made any conscious connection at this stage. Chloe tended to organise things in lines and watch the movement of the wheels on her brother's cars go back and forth. She would lie flat on the floor and could be there for what seemed like

Discovery

hours. This played out in the assessment as well. Other things were noted but by then my mind, brain and heart had aligned on the fact that I was about to jump in and land in this world of autism.

As the assessment finished Dr Oliver moved over to speak with us, her tone kind and at the same time being very clear. She said that her conclusion was that Chloe was displaying signs of autism and it was her view that we should ensure that she got access to the right support and guidance to help her over the next couple of years prior to her starting school. We asked about the 'Statementing' process (the now labelled Educational Health Care Plan aka EHCP) and she said it was very rare for local authorities to provide a statement of needs to pre-school age children but that she would absolutely support our efforts to get this done. What followed was a pack of documents full of guidance, advice and places to go to for support. Looking back, I remember feeling numb, like I had somehow been responsible for Chloe's condition. Had I caused it via the pregnancy? Was the polyhydramnios responsible? Was the VSD a sign? Could they have picked it up when she was in my stomach and helped? Had my fear of operations and instead electing for a natural delivery been the cause of her coming out with the cord around her neck (contrary to the option of a C-section as offered by the consultant)?

Bigger Than the Moon

If it had not been around her neck, would she have been okay? Was it the significant emotional stress I had experienced during the pregnancy as a result of the personal issues I had gone through? Was it because I worked really hard? Was it because I was not happy? Should I have done anything different? Was it something I ate? The questions went on and on in my head and even now they come and go – they stay for a lot less time, however. I have learnt over the years to be kind to myself.

I did feel a sense of relief. My body and mind became less heavy, less confused. I gained a sense of clarity. I also gained a sense of purpose. How important is purpose to the human journey? Chloe's diagnosis allowed me to name 'it'. Naming conventions are important. It's not that the label becomes the point, but it provides you with a key to access sources of information and support and gives you a place to start. It's the beginning of a long process and can, if you are up for it, spring you into action so you can understand what you are going to need to help you and manage the prognosis.

Chloe's diagnosis was formally confirmed in November 2011. Up until this point, labelling my child with a special need would have been a terrible idea to me, the high-performing, high-achieving individual who did everything to perfection (or so I thought). This world I had found myself

Discovery

in was not my view of perfection (or so I thought.) Then I began to ask hard questions of myself: 'Was this the lesson I had to learn?' Had my quest and drive for 'perfection' landed me where I was right now in terms of my personal life? Had I been seeing things in the wrong way? Was this the time for me to see perfection in a different way? I felt as if I was about to find out what life was really all about. I started to feel strangely liberated with Chloe's diagnosis. I drew on my love for learning and natural curiosity to understand things I did not know. This was new territory for me, and I was ready to learn, understand and go into this new place life was leading me to.

So 2011 was a year of disruption, discovery and movement. A place where I jolted from one level to another. I voraciously read any book I could about autism; you name it, I read it. Books written by parents who felt they had the keys to 'curing' their child's autism, books from people whose life's work was to observe the condition and provide sources of help and information to manage it. For a while I also explored the field of Advanced Behavioural Analysis (aka ABA) and attended a seminar from an organisation where I must have purchased about five huge A4-size books from potty training (Chloe was still very much in pull-ups and would be until just before she started school) to how to prepare for school and interacting with other

Bigger Than the Moon

children and teachers. This seminar filled my head with all the things I would need to consider, manage and most importantly pay for (which was basically the point of the seminar if the truth be told) in order to ensure a successful future for my child, who, without this therapy, would be lost. I left feeling scared, which did not feel right to me. Weren't these types of forums meant to make you feel helped? I was therefore slightly cynical but still not fully in the driving seat of this new situation so I questioned my judgement and therefore deferred to these 'expert' forums for help to construct my path. In essence I lost my intuition for a while and leaned less on it and more on the external environment for my cues and direction. I approached this situation as I would with a work project: to build knowledge, find the right experts to help you and apply the learning. If only it was that simple. Fear is a powerful thing, and whilst it can propel you and move you forward it can also paralyze you and, if not managed, make you doubt yourself. It's the thing to master so you can use it in the right way.

I would eventually let go of my need to read about all things autism. It was a deeply personal choice. I felt the more I read books on what to do and how to manage the diagnosis and the multitude of interventions, I was losing focus on what was right for Chloe. The first thing

Discovery

anyone will tell you who is well-versed in this topic is how autism is a spectrum and everyone on it is different. I realised that the knowledge I needed to discover was in Chloe first and foremost. I also came to the awareness that in order to be in the best possible position to help Chloe I couldn't be drained from reading about all possible therapies, interventions and sometimes very contradictory views on how to deal with autism. I had to help Chloe, but I also had to have energy for other parts of my life too. I made the decision quite early in this process to learn as I worked with Chloe to support her. She would be my guide.

In December 2011, I began a mini campaign of sorts: 'The Plan for Chloe'. I was predicting a bumpy road ahead for us in the effort to get Chloe the support she needed in the nursery (even with the diagnosis confirmed), as well as trying to get her an official Statement of Needs which would be a legal and statutory process obliging the local authority to provide specific support to Chloe in her educational development and to ensure all her needs could and would be met. So I decided to alert the highest levels of office to the situation with my little girl. Anyone who knows me will not be surprised by any of this; I have this innate sense of right and wrong and am the first to pick up the lead, take charge and start a movement! I decided,

Bigger Than the Moon

even though nothing technically had gone wrong – yet – I would get in front of the situation by contacting my local MP, Department for Education and even the Prime Minister's office about Chloe's needs. If nothing else, I figured that when the process did kick off, Chloe's name would already be known and so would mine (with a red flag attached to it no doubt).

I sent my first letter to the local authority executive at the time. I decided that these letters would be genuine and authentic attempts to solicit help and support for my plan for Chloe. I adopted a more human approach and tone, as opposed to just a plain request for help with an issue and not really focusing on who it was for. I would attach to the email (or physically if hard copy) a picture of Chloe so they knew that this was about a person, a very little one, and that I was advocating on her behalf. The letter was heartfelt and sincere but very certain that I would do whatever was necessary to get the help that Chloe needed. I sent a copy of that letter to my MP, who was very visible in their advocacy of special needs issues and was known to be responsive and proactive in providing support (and did not disappoint).

To round it off nicely I also sent a letter to the Prime Minister's office. I did not expect a response – I think it just made me feel like I was doing my best and whatever I could

Discovery

to fight for Chloe. I did get a response from the office, however, dated 20 December 2011, and I have kept that letter to this day. It was a polite acknowledgement of my letter and said they had forwarded on my concerns to the Department for Health and the Department for Education. I also got a response from both those departments as well, who subsequently outlined the Special Educational Needs (SEN) process to me and explained that the local authority would be responsible for processing this application. None of this information was a surprise and was expected: the aim was to raise awareness and visibility and ensure that my local authority understood the seriousness of Chloe's situation and could see that a protracted SEN assessment process would only exacerbate an already negative experience that Chloe was going through and therefore this needed to be accelerated. The executive head of the local authority did respond via the head of the SEN team to confirm that they would be in touch regarding the SEN process. There was a very short space of time between my initial letters and then the final response. I would come to learn the importance of raising matters quickly, urgently and in parallel. Don't sit and wait and believe the system is going to automatically help you.

At this stage, I began to feel overwhelmed. One day at work I was in my office with the door closed and a

Bigger Than the Moon

colleague of mine, Gemma, peeked through the window and knocked to come in. We had become firm friends and healthy competitors, having started at Citi in the same team within the same year (she joined just before me.) We were aligned as newbies, in a very long-service institution, to bring new ideas and thinking to life in a strong culture (and we managed to change a lot whilst we were there). Gemma had an uncanny sense of sniffing out when something was not right.

As she walked into my office, I remember having tears in my eyes and saying, 'Chloe has been diagnosed with autism.' Saying it out loud to her made it feel real, like something I could hold and define. It was the first time I had said this at work. She looked at me and what followed was the start of a bond that was to last for the time we were at Citi together and beyond, to this day. She did what was natural to her; she came to where I was sitting at my desk and gave me a hug. She then sat down opposite me and said the magic words, 'How can I help you right now?' It was typical Gemma and she just knew what I needed to hear at the time. There were no other questions about the situation, just a genuine desire to help me through that moment, and I will never forget the kindness she showed me then and still does. The ability to share your challenges with people at work who you spend most of your time

Discovery

with is important (and I know this is not always possible). It allows them to know that there is more to you than just what appears on the surface, and whilst you don't have to over-share it helps for people to see the human in you. This was something I learned the value of more as the years went by, especially with the teams I managed.

You have to remember that my world was like being in the storm during this time: everything was happening at once and I still needed to function for both my children. Che was struggling at school and more than once I had to remind the school, when they too wanted to tell me he had 'had a bad day', that his whole world had been turned upside down since his parents separated and what he needed at school was support, space and understanding, rather than reports of apparent disruptive behaviour sent home to his parents via a book. Che was a sensitive child who felt the loss of his mum and dad being together intensely. We were a close unit and did most things together – this was a new operating model for him and he needed a lot of support during this time to cope with his 'new normal'. He was eight years old and, unlike Chloe, his age did not protect him from the realisation of what this meant. Both his dad and I kept to a routine and provided a consistency and stability that mitigated the sense of loss as much as we could. The school eventually responded in the right way and things began to improve.

As my role developed, my work required that I travel in manageable chunks, mainly to New York but also across the EMEA region. These trips had also become a space for me to rediscover me. I let go and learnt to love myself by myself, although it took a while for this to be fully felt. I would take the time after a day full of meetings to go out in NYC and buy myself things, eat at nice places, visit art galleries, and take in the sights, sounds and smells. NYC is an amazing city and I credit it with allowing me to rediscover who Syreeta was and could be during this time. It was less about the experiences themselves and more about taking myself out and being by myself whilst having them. I realised that caring for myself was going to be important if I wanted to be in a strong position to support Chloe and Che. It was not just a physical strength that would be required but more an emotional one. Being alone was important and getting comfortable with that in a good way would be invaluable as I moved forward.

New York had always been a familiar place to me with many family members living there, and my grandmother lived most of the latter part of her life there as a nurse. She had moved there when her children were still young. Her reason was to be able to earn enough money for a better

Discovery

life for all of them (a familiar story and a repeat of her leaving my mother and her sister (my aunt), in Jamaica – although they were much younger at three and two respectively). I often wonder if NYC was an escape for her too, albeit she made it a much more permanent one and was to be there for some twenty years, returning every year to see family. She had also 'escaped' Jamaica. Hers was a familiar story in Caribbean and African culture: the pattern of leaving and returning and children caught up in the middle; some faring better than others.

Now, however, going through my own journey of discovery and change, it felt like I was experiencing the feeling of escape my grandmother may have felt when she arrived in this unique part of America. New York is a wonderful place for the senses to be awakened and aligned. The general feeling I had at the time was that I was indeed being jolted into a new reality and leaving another behind. It, too, felt like an 'escape' for the time I was there, although I never wanted to make it permanent and the thought of leaving my children behind never crossed my mind. Maybe this was because it was different times, or maybe I was just going to break the cycle of what had tended to happen with those before me. Having these moments to be on my own served as much-needed respite and a time to refuel. This would be essential for

Bigger Than the Moon

the road I knew I had to travel to get Chloe the help she needed as well as to support Che and manage my work schedule.

That being said, all of this change and disruption was also very tiring. I would always make sure as far as I could that my work trips would be timed around the two nights in the week that their dad would have them – so I managed to do very quick trips over two to three days and return straight into the childcare routine. It was tough going, given the change in time zones, and I had to be prepared to be effective at work, whilst feeling completely exhausted. However, it is amazing how the body and mind adjust to new levels of endurance, creating a new normal. I could feel myself evolving as if preparing for a marathon. However, the race had already started: I was in it now and there was no going back. During this period I also sought guidance and support to help me process what was happening to me in order to be able to function effectively for myself and my children. There is only so much self-care work you can do on your own.

Mountains

Setting off on the journey of discovery for Chloe led me to places I had not foreseen and had not planned for but in many ways, through this process, new doors were opening despite this being a very hard time for me. Towards the end of 2011, I had started to work for somebody new (who had been away on maternity leave when I joined Citi and hence why the lovely Daryl was managing me for a while – he and I now became peers). As part of the annual performance review, I was informed that I had received a promotion. I knew I had worked hard and delivered beyond what was expected; however, I was not expecting to hear this news. I was given a letter and my new manager smiled and then said, 'Congratulations, this promotion is so well deserved!'

I felt a bit stumped. I was just happy to be in work and be able to survive financially. The promotion was completely unexpected, although as I started to reflect on what I had achieved in the last year, it felt as if I deserved it. I remember being overcome with emotions. I had decided not to tell anyone about what was happening to me personally beyond Daryl and Gemma. For me work was a refuge; it was the one part of my world during that time that I felt I could control and determine. I could also forget for a few hours (barring the odd call from my lawyer, the nursery and the school that interrupted the calm intermittently!). It was therefore a place of high productivity and I enjoyed being able to continue to nurture this part of my life.

As the year continued it was clear that the challenges with Chloe's nursery were not abating. They had started to get more insistent that Chloe needed extra support in the setting (and they would always be at pains to stress that this was not to be funded by them). Sometimes I would pick her up and she would be the happiest child. This would most often be when the day had gone according to her likes and preferences. If it had been a bad day it would have been because there was some form of disruption or change. Other times it would be that an interaction with another child had not gone well.

It was so hard for me as her parent: Chloe now had an officially diagnosed need and effectively was registered disabled as a result, but hidden disabilities don't get the instant recognition, tolerance and empathy that can accompany a physical one. I wanted there to be more tolerance and understanding from staff as well as parents.

Mountains

On the other hand, I could also empathise with how staff and other parents were feeling, knowing how increasingly hard it was becoming to manage Chloe at home, and if it were my child being impacted, I likely would have felt the same as they did when they complained to the nursery. It hurt me deeply as I knew that the behaviour was a direct result of the condition she had been diagnosed with as opposed to her being 'naughty'. The feedback abated for a while, then would come back as soon as Chloe's routine was affected, or she was tired or became overwhelmed (sensory processing disorder is a big part of how autism affects her). The noise, sights and sounds of a busy nursery environment did not align well for Chloe, especially towards the end of the day when she would be physically exhausted.

My mini campaign of sorts called 'The Plan for Chloe' continued. Chloe had been under one local authority from a residential perspective but in another one for the location of her nursery, as we lived on the border between the two. This was a very complex process and it took a herculean effort to send email after email and letter after letter to various teams to get them to connect and talk. As Chloe had a registered disability this was very helpful as there were legal and statutory requirements that everyone was obliged to observe. But nobody made it easy. I was

Bigger Than the Moon

also going through the SEN process, the aim of which would be to provide a statement of her needs. This was going to be invaluable in the effort to get the right level of attention and focus for what Chloe needed; without it she would be lost in the system at best and at worst, as with so many children like Chloe, forgotten. To be forgotten means you may never be found. Case workers move around often and handovers are sometimes not as effective as they can be, so it can be very demanding on a parent's time and energy to make sure they stay on top of things and ahead of any changes. So many parents I have spoken to often believe what they are told the first time and become misguided about getting the right support for their children early enough and think the system will work without their constant oversight, which in my experience is rarely the case.

I was very fortunate to be introduced to the National Autistic Society (NAS) EarlyBird programme for parents as part of the diagnosis support. I had applied to get on the programme that was due to commence in the March of the same year. There was a delay as it became threatened with closure due to a 'lack of funding'. How many times would I hear that phrase over the next few years! Rarely deterred, I sent a letter to the council and then to my local MP to challenge this (luckily a few other parents

Mountains

had done the same) and after some effort they confirmed the programme would go ahead.

If you know that your child needs more support or you need support to help them, it's important to always fight and challenge. It's hard work but often it is what is needed to open the door that may seem closed. If you don't know how to do this, seek out those who do. Contact your local MP, contact the Citizens Advice Bureau and, if you have the means, speak to a law firm specialising in Special Educational Needs.

This programme would also introduce me to fellow warrior parents and one person in particular, Natalie, became a friend and invaluable support to me over the years and to this day in the various situations I find myself having to navigate with Chloe.

Natalie was a trojan. A 'force multiplier' as Colin Powell would say. I was instantly drawn to her and the energy she exuded and identified with her 'no-nonsense' attitude. I have always been a humble learner, eager to understand and be curious about things I don't know. I leaned into Natalie and found ways through this wood I found myself in – she cleared paths for me that I don't even think she realised she did. She helped me to understand how to navigate getting support that Chloe would be entitled to, as well as the process of registering Chloe as disabled.

Bigger Than the Moon

This was a new world to me and I had assumed things would happen automatically. It was a rude awakening to find that I had to seek out what Chloe was entitled to and be persistent when everything seemed to require me to 'make a case' to justify why. It made me wonder about all those parents who did not have access to support and people like Natalie, who manage the myriad of unwritten rules in this world of special needs. I got a lot of energy from Natalie in those early days and she kept me going. I am forever grateful for her and many like her who came to help me.

I was always impressed with these warrior women who I met in that group. We all had varying experiences with our children and came from very diverse backgrounds, but one thing was consistent; we were laser-focused on ensuring that our children had the best support, be it from us or other agencies. I found this group became the beginning of an informal network I would tap into to get valuable advice and guidance. I was sometimes frustrated that I did not have time to engage with many of them as regularly as I would have liked. Many of the parents were full-time carers. They had made the decision to do so for their child/children because of their needs. I was acutely aware that in many jobs/professions it is not possible to accommodate the flexibility that is required for

Mountains

the various appointments and meetings that flood your calendar when you have a child with special needs. I do wonder how much more support I would have gained if I'd had the opportunity to engage more with the group and benefit from their experience. It does make a difference when you are around people who truly understand your world and live it every day. But I would end up building my own version of the group as time went on, in different ways and discovering more people who were in a similar position to me, as my journey continued.

Whilst I sometimes saw my professional seniority as a burden when it came to managing Chloe, it was also a blessing given the flexibility I was able to employ in navigating the various schedules of both my children as well as perform well in my work.

As part of the review of Chloe's situation at the nursery the local authority moved very quickly to understand whether Chloe could attend a specialist local authority pre-school nursery, which had an Autism Spectrum Disorder (ASD) unit, as part of the SEN assessment process. These were very rare but there was a good one led by an amazing individual with a great team. As you would expect, places for this provision were scarce. We would very quickly need to arrange an educational psychologist assessment and this was facilitated by the local authority, given the circumstances of Chloe's situation with the private day nursery, which had now been escalated as an urgent matter to resolve.

The assessment was held in a building that served as a unit for children's educational needs services. I remember the psychologist being fascinated with Chloe (as most people were and continue to be). I did my normal recount of her story, background, health history and my own observations as her parent. I was now an expert in this narrative and was able to talk fluently through this. This was no doubt aided by my work in HR and business in which you never had much time to get a lot of information across. After many questions and answers, as well as observing her in play, the psychologist came to the conclusion that a specialist nursery would be helpful and, more importantly, vital for Chloe. Given she was likely to receive a SEN statement there was also a strong possibility that she could secure a place, albeit that places were tight. He said that she was 'a very special young girl'. She had (still has) this ability to give out an energy without saying anything and normally just through a smile. I will always remember his words and have heard them many times since from other people when talking about Chloe.

Chloe managed to get a part-time place at the local authority nursery so would attend the provision for the

Mountains

morning and then get transport back to the private nursery for the rest of the day. We believed that with this additional support, it would ease some of the challenges being experienced in the private nursery setting and reduce her time there (and by default ease the pressure on their resources, which was their primary concern). Her escort for the transport was James. James was just the most pleasant person you could meet, who had extensive experience with children with disabilities and made both her dad and I feel secure and confident about leaving our little three-year-old to get in a mid-size bus with him and other children. Either her dad or I would pick her up after work, depending on who she was due to be with. Again, all of this support and provision was made possible by the focus and attention we were receiving from the family support team at the local authority. It is important to emphasise that there were some good people who helped us and we were grateful for their commitment to making sure this situation was worked through to the right conclusion. I often wonder what Chloe's story would have been if she had not got the right support in place early. Another statistic perhaps? Undiagnosed or misdiagnosed with a label that pointed more towards 'behavioural issues' as opposed to a stated disability. This has become the fate of so many young people who are victims of a system that fails to recognise their true needs early enough, if at all.

In 2012, whilst managing the back and forth between the nursery and local authorities, I was finalising the financial settlement as part of the divorce arrangements. The summer of 2012 marked the beginning of my process to self-heal and self-love whilst continuing to fight for my little girl and learning how to co-parent. During this time I was constantly supported by my best friend Susan. Susan was also Chloe's godmother and completely devoted to her as well as to Che. She came and rescued me at a time when I did not realise that I needed to be rescued; silently she would show up to my home unprompted and lie down next to me and we would chat forever, laugh and also be present in moments where I felt I could not keep going. She is the kind of best friend that a person who finds it hard to be vulnerable needs. Susan moved with my emotions and sat with them rather than fight them away, but at the same time she helped me to be aware of those emotions and acknowledge them and she worked with me as I figured out how to overcome them. She understood the mountain I was climbing and decided she would climb it with me, but she never announced this; instead she moved with actions and unspoken sentiments. I will never forget how she showed up during this time.

Mountains

We had decided that in the summer of 2012 we would go on a trip to Jamaica with our children. We were booked into an all-inclusive hotel in Montego Bay on the north coast. Chloe was three and a half and Che was nine. Susan's son Kyle was twelve. What a magical holiday. The process of 'returning' is so important, and for me Jamaica was my place of return – not just physically but also mentally and spiritually. It was after all the birthplace of my parents and I was lucky enough to be able to know it well, having been taken there a few times by my parents as a child for very long and wonderful holidays. We would go with my uncle and aunt and my cousins and there was one trip together with my grandparents on my dad's side (a special holiday). So it really did feel like home for me. I grew up in a distinctly Caribbean household back in the UK, so culturally this was more familiar than the feeling of being just British: as a young child growing up in the 80s and the experiences that went with that, Jamaica was a contrast as I never felt rejected there or was made to feel 'different'. It welcomed me with warmth. I felt like Syreeta there and not defined by the colour of my skin as with so many experiences I had as a child in the marginal world I was placed in back in the UK. It was liberating as a child and would continue to be on every visit. I am grateful my parents worked hard to introduce me to their

Bigger Than the Moon

homeland early in my life, so I knew there was another place that was also home and made me feel seen in a positive way. I wanted the same for my children, especially Chloe, so that they knew this feeling too.

Taking my children to Jamaica therefore was a continuation of this legacy – it was not Che's first trip to Jamaica but it was Chloe's. The holiday proved to be much-needed therapy for me and provided a brief respite from the reality awaiting me back home. Chloe's challenges continued to come alive for me during this break, however. Firstly, her need for routine was becoming more and more pronounced. She would become distressed if her schedule changed in any way. Patterns were important for Chloe. There was an elevator at the hotel that she particularly liked being wheeled into in her buggy. If this elevator looked full of people as the doors opened she would start screaming and not want to be wheeled in. We had to wait until an empty one arrived which proved difficult at busy periods.

It was so nice being on holiday with Susan and Kyle, who intuitively got that a holiday with Chloe meant adapting a lot! They did so with patience, love and understanding. Che was a veteran in this space and would always work with me to figure out how we could manage these situations as they arose. The stares from other

Mountains

people watching Chloe's meltdowns did not faze him, even though I know it affected him; he was only nine after all. However, his love for Chloe meant he always put her first. Once we knew what affected her, we would establish a contingency and that would become our routine. For the elevator scenario, we found a very under-utilised one at the far end of our hotel and so that became 'Chloe's elevator' – problem solved!

Travelling with children always requires good planning if you want a holiday to go smoothly. Travelling with a child with autism requires more maniacal planning than you could ever imagine; if you want it to at least feel like a form of a holiday going smoothly is a bonus. It was important to me to meet this challenge for a number of reasons:

1. I knew that I could if I tried hard enough.
2. I believed that Chloe should be able to access the same opportunities that I was able to give Che. I did not want her 'disability' to mean that she somehow became disabled from experiencing life.
3. Chloe was young enough for me to be able to influence how she could learn to adapt and manage different situations. Whilst she had started to develop rigid routines and schedules

for herself, I wanted her to also understand how to manage changes and different situations; and begin to process how change could be a part of a routine as well. This is why I am such a firm advocate for early intervention in the diagnosis of autism.

4. Finally, holidays were important to me! I wanted to see if I could continue to enjoy a part of my life that I valued in spite of the challenges presented by managing autism. It is so easy to become a defeatist when faced with something that appears to put barriers in your way. Your mindset is extremely important.

That being said it was still very hard to do, as well as physically and emotionally draining. Firstly I had to think through the airport; managing Chloe and Che through security and making sure I could physically support her, the buggy, Che, our luggage and figure out how to make sure she did not become overwhelmed. Noises, especially kids screaming, and the chaos of a queue were instant triggers for Chloe (and remain so): she could go from calm to hysterical in minutes, sometimes seconds. I always knew the signs – a sudden focus or her attention directed to the source of the trigger and a small moment of calm before

Mountains

an overwhelming storm. One that could last seconds or long minutes that would drain both me and her, as well as cause silent distress for Che, although he never admitted it. I could sense it, however. He was a sensitive soul and never expressed his emotions easily. He was always very considerate of Chloe and in a way, I think, also of me. His way of helping was to not appear too disrupted.

Another important consideration when travelling was managing Chloe in environments that were dramatically different and created very significant sounds for her. The gangway to a plane entrance door, for example, the plane itself as well as the varying and loud noises of a toilet on the plane. Chloe did not do well in public toilets generally (although she was still in nappies at this point, on the longest road to potty training! Oh the Pampers and Pull-Ups we went through!). She was terrified of entering a public toilet as a result of the noise of a dryer. It's hard to really explain how much fear and pain there is in certain sounds for children with sensory processing needs; they are highly sensitised and it can be hard to watch and manage when your child is clearly in distress because of something that does not seem to have any effect on you. It's amazing how insignificant processes like drying your hands after going to the toilet become major tasks to think through when managing a disability like autism. It requires significant preparation and planning. Enter the magic solution: hand sanitiser and ear defenders!

Another magic solution was the iPad. Steve Jobs may not have been thinking of autistic children when working with his team to design this device, but I think his own tendencies and ways of thinking aligned well. It became a magical device for Chloe before I saw the trend that this really could help neurodivergent people engage, communicate and connect better. Chloe's gross and fine motor skill challenges became less so with her hands being able to move the visual on the screen effortlessly and her sensory processing worked much more effectively. Much of her learning has been accelerated by the digital learning age and I for one am very grateful to the Jobs and Jony Ives of this world. These things made travelling manageable and reduced the trauma of the odd meltdown. I also ensured I spoke with the airline in advance of travelling to ensure they were aware that Chloe had autism and that we had time to priority board and settle Chloe in to her seat and get familiar without having to navigate a long queue. This was way before the increased levels of autism awareness we have today in airports and on planes, but even back then some airlines were familiar once approached and did help me. It is important to note that I had already travelled with Chloe and Che on a plane, but on those occasions

Mountains

there had been two of us to handle things and she was still a baby, not yet manifesting the visible behavioural signs of autism – she was still in the 'quiet' and 'observing' stage then so we did not have to manage things in the way I had to when she was a bit older and I was a solo travelling parent!

On this trip to Jamaica I did have my best friend Susan, however, who continued her love affair with Chloe at a deeper level, given we were effectively living together over the two-week period. She got to understand Chloe better and was curious to get to know more about her world. I believe this is why Chloe responded to Susan in a way that I had only seen her do with her dad, brother and myself. It made things that little bit easier for me on the holiday, having someone else who could be with Chloe quite comfortably and confidently.

One day we went on a trip to Negril beach, and during lunch I became more aware of what impact it had on Chloe when she became overwhelmed. If she was tired, hot or unclear about what was happening her face would quickly betray how she was feeling inside. There would be a look of confusion and frustration because she was unable to say what was wrong or articulate what she wanted. My ability to help Chloe though these moments went beyond just a verbal or physical interaction. I had to learn to be patient

Bigger Than the Moon

and work with her, even through some very loud and quite extreme meltdowns, and try to 'hear' what she wanted to tell me but just couldn't. It would be one of the things that I found so difficult to manage with Chloe's autism. I could not always instantly get what she wanted and she could not tell me how she was feeling or what was wrong with her. Helplessness is the most devastating feeling a parent can have; however, I learned to hone the intuitive understanding in our relationship and connect on a level that did not require words or communication. We learned by just looking at each other or by me reaching for her hand and just letting her know I was there. It became a magical language I would come to treasure.

On this holiday Susan and I also became very aware of how in tune Chloe was with her environment and the world in a positive way and not just in the challenges of managing her sensory processing needs. Being around Chloe meant being very present; and watching her on this holiday was our favourite pastime, which remains to this day. She would hate walking with shoes on and insisted on being barefoot (still does). Chloe was not afraid of insects (unlike her brother) and would watch them with curiosity, happy to pick one up and turn her head to examine it. She would stop and look at flowers or be aware of the wind moving the leaves in the trees.

Mountains

At night she and I would look up at the stars (a favourite activity of mine) and we would observe the moon in the clear night sky of the Caribbean. It was on this holiday that we began our ritual, which lasts to this day, of me asking her how much she loved me, and she in response would say, 'This much', holding her little arms and hands out wide. I would then follow up and say, 'How much?' and point towards the moon. She would quickly reply, 'Bigger than the moon and back!' and we would both laugh and hug each other. I have always made sure that both my children look up at the sky and notice the different phases of the moon. It is a wonderfully powerful force that is bigger than we can imagine; it seems fitting that it became a symbol of the love and connection I have with both of them. It was helping Chloe connect with the idea that the love we shared was indeed bigger than the moon.

☾

It was August 2012 when we returned from holiday and back to the mad grind of what was then my life: managing the children, work (lots of changes were taking place at work during this time. I was about to change bosses, jobs, and restructure my team), nursery and the various school and extra-curricular activities for Che (there were many!). I was also struggling to understand the changes I was going through in my life. Sometimes I would wake up and be confused as to where I had got to. It felt like I was receiving mixed signals from the universe: two beautiful children and one ex-husband, an amazing job but incredibly challenging work and long hours, friends arriving and friends disappearing and a few constant ones, and managing the financial burden of keeping the world turning for myself and my children. There were moments of exhilaration as well as complete devastation and despair. A key lesson for me throughout was the sense that I had to keep holding on. I could not just give up as I had the sense it would get better if I stuck with it and I would turn that metaphorical corner. But there were times when I wanted to stop. I learnt to find ways to explore these moments, either through journalling, travelling or leaning into my creative side. I realised that you could change your perspective on something, even in the most challenging moments. Always ask yourself 'What's the upside?' – seek it out and believe there is something that you can benefit from in times where all seems lost. It's the 'dark wood', the 'selva oscura' Dante talks about, and it is necessary in order to understand and benefit from the good that is eventually found in the journey.

Mountains

But then the journey through my dark wood seemed to pause in this part of my life one evening when I returned from work. I had a note from Royal Mail noting a letter that needed to be signed for at my local sorting office. It was dark and raining and one of the evenings my children were with their dad. I was shattered and exhausted from work but I made my way to the sorting office and collected the letter. That evening is so vivid to me, even now. A sense of foreboding came over me as at this point in my life I seemed to be managing so much unexpected news and felt the letter had to be important for me to have to sign for it. I did not wait to get into the car to open it. Standing outside with the rain coming down on me and feeling cold, I opened the letter with trepidation and my heart beating so much it felt like I could hear it. It was a letter from the nursery Chloe attended. Its main objective? To tell me my little girl was being excluded from the nursery. I can recall the tears falling down my face in the same way as the tiny rain droplets, slowly becoming indistinguishable from each other as both cascaded down.

Descent

Recalling the events that followed is a painful and confusing process and sometimes it is hard to piece all the moments together; the calls, the emails, the meetings, still going to work and dealing with all kinds of things there, and the agonising over what was best for Chloe. It felt like such a cruel thing to do to her and the stress it placed on me was enormous. Childcare was a critical part of my ability to be able to work and continue to support my home and children and basically keep functioning. I worked full-time and managed to keep everything going in a very senior role due to the composition of support for my children, which basically was their dad, me, nursery and after-school club for Che plus a forward-thinking employer that supported flexible working. Nobody else helped us or indeed offered to or asked if we needed any help.

It was not a case of just finding another place for Chloe; she now had a diagnosed disability and specific special needs and could not 'just' go anywhere, and any

Descent

care provision had to be carefully thought through. I did not have family on my side who could help as everybody worked themselves. It felt like I was at an impasse.

Once the local authority were made aware of the exclusion letter, an urgent meeting was called between them and the nursery. It was acknowledged that the nursery could not just exclude Chloe on the grounds of her disability as there were statutory and legal obligations that needed to be observed, but neither were they obliged to continue to support Chloe without appropriate funding. It made me feel vindicated that I fought to get her diagnosed as early as I did, as it was the thing that was now helping me to get the right attention on Chloe's situation.

However, an event at nursery towards the end of the year as Christmas approached, prompted me to stop rationalising and thinking logically but listen to what my heart was telling me. I went to pick Chloe up one day as usual after work. I was greeted by looks of concern and the familiar face I had come to recognise which normally preceded me being told that 'Chloe has had a bad day'. As I walked into the room, I looked over to where Chloe was and saw my little girl with her small frame and helpless face, looking completely shattered sitting at the little table for the children. She was silent but clearly distressed, with her head in her hands, almost using them like a cradle.

Bigger Than the Moon

She looked up at me with a pleading expression and her cheeks were marked white from old tears that had stained her face, which suggested she had been crying for a very long time. She was clearly shattered and exhausted from her latest meltdown. This time, however, Chloe looked like she had reached the end of the road, as if staying one more day at the nursery would be too much. She did not have to say anything to me to tell me how she felt. I could feel my breath pause in what was just pure shock (and anger) at how she looked.

The thing that most impacted me about that scene was how alone Chloe was. Nobody was with her. She looked physically and mentally isolated. I knew I had to act, and as much as I wanted to fight for her to be treated fairly in her nursery setting, I also had to accept that this was no longer a healthy environment for Chloe and did not serve her. I went over to my baby girl and she instantly reached for me and just put her head on my chest. I met her face as she leaned in and whispered in her ears, 'It's okay, Chloe, Mummy is going to take care of you.' She remained silent.

I had no words for the nursery staff who were talking to me all the time throughout this scene, attempting to explain the reasons behind what I was seeing, but whose words were muted to my ears. My whole focus and attention was on Chloe. I silently picked up her bags and the

Descent

belongings she had at the nursery, all the time still holding her tightly to me so she felt secure, and ignored all sounds from the manager. I just looked at them knowing that this would be the last time Chloe would be at the nursery. I wanted to cry but held all the tears back, knowing how many Chloe had cried already; she needed to feel reassured and know that everything was okay. As I stepped out of the nursery and made my way to the car, I called her dad and said to him, 'She is never going back there. I don't know how we will sort out new childcare and what will happen with work, but Chloe is never going back to that nursery.' He agreed.

Mastering your ego is a continuous process. At this point I needed to master mine and ensure that in my effort to get her the right support and make the nursery be accountable (and in some ways for me to be 'proved right'), I did not need to do this at the expense of Chloe's mental health and well-being. I had to balance my fight to make the nursery and local authority do the right thing with ensuring she was safe and her well-being was prioritised. She had to leave immediately, and I had to find another solution and another way.

Angels

Just as the descent took an accelerated pace into unknown territory for Chloe and me, people started to turn up in our lives to help manage the fall. I had not planned their arrival and did not even seek them out. But just by making the decision to take Chloe out of what was becoming an intolerable situation, it seemed the universe responded with an equivalent action and sent people to help me. The timing of the decision coincided with my impending Christmas holiday booked from work. This meant that I could cover Chloe's childcare needs together with her dad whilst we figured out what we would do. Learning to be brave and bold when you don't have the answers is so important. It was a lesson I learnt from my work in managing and leading teams, and it was becoming more of a lesson in my personal life.

In the meanwhile the family services team came to see me. They were equally shocked at what we had experienced and sympathetic to the situation. I made it clear that

Angels

it was not my intention to send her back and we needed to work through a plan B. They sat down with me at my home and gave me a list of potential childminders, all of whom had some form of expertise/experience of working with children with special needs. I must admit at this point it was clear to anyone who took the time to be with me that I had reached a point of surrender (in a bad way). I did not have anything left in me, or so I thought. Seeing my daughter in such a distressed state really impacted me and this team stepped in at a very crucial time to help me. I could not see a way out and they helped me to understand my options and potential ways to find a solution. I will always appreciate the help they provided: yes, it was their job but I also believed they genuinely cared and were determined to help find a solution for Chloe.

I looked down at the various names, addresses and contact details. My eyes seemed to land on one in particular: Claire. I didn't know why I was drawn to this particular name. Perhaps it was because her address was one of the closest to mine. I mentioned her name to the team, who gave me the background and said that Claire was a very warm individual who had a lot of experience with a range of children. She had been a childminder for a long time and the team knew her quite well from other referrals. She was one of three names I circled; however, hers would be the only telephone number I would need to ring.

I went to visit Claire shortly after and as soon as she opened the door, Chloe walked straight in almost as if she had been there before, and I was immediately struck by a sense of warmth and understanding. We talked about Chloe, what had happened and her needs. The one thing I remember from this initial interaction is that Claire did not assume anything. She wanted to understand Chloe, so most of her questions focused on that. She gave me a sense that we would work together to figure things out. I liked her style and approach and believed it was what Chloe needed – someone with no expectations but with absolute hope for the way forward.

Chloe started with Claire in January 2013 and she would remain her childminder for nearly eight years. Her transport arrangements, which had been in place from her time at the ASD unit, would continue but instead of dropping her at the private nursery, Chloe would be dropped off at Claire's. Her escort would continue to be James, who had been with her since she first started to receive transport assistance. When she first started going on transport, she seemed to be too tiny to be going off on her own in what looked like a big coach (it was more of a Transit van

Angels

size!) and although other kids were with her, as a parent it was the most devastating feeling watching your little child, only three and a half years old, go off without you. Chloe had a fortitude and confidence about her, however, that made me feel confident and assured, even in these moments of doubt.

I remember the first time she went on transport from her dad's house. I got up early and made my way over to his house and waited outside. Her dad came out with Chloe and her brother, and she was smiling as she saw me. She looked a bit confused as this was not the normal routine, me showing up or indeed James coming to take her to a new place. We introduced her to James, who she took to immediately. He helped to lift her on the steps into the bus and she marched towards her seat with that distinctive walk of hers and sat on the seat smiling at us through the window. It was at these moments that I realised more and more that Chloe was actually helping me. I had to conquer my fear that this autism world would be a permanent thing for my daughter, but it seemed she was rolling with it. Why wouldn't she? This was her world and perfectly normal for her; the lesson for me was how to make it normal for myself and others who would need to engage and be with her. I was moving slowly towards acceptance of this new world step by step.

Bigger Than the Moon

James also made time to talk to Che. He would ensure that Che was acknowledged and included when talking to us in the pick-up process and he got to learn about Che and his likes and dislikes. Siblings of children with special needs also require as much attention as they do. Their world is impacted beyond belief and it is essential to never neglect their needs (knowingly or unknowingly), which can sometimes happen in the whirlwind that surrounds the world of SEN. James's acts of kindness to both Chloe and Che will stay with me forever. He would remain Chloe's transport escort for a while – in fact until Chloe went to primary school.

Chloe continued at the ASD nursery unit and seemed to be developing well. The nursery also supported her potty training, which was a slow process but moving in the right direction. I continued to observe the differences I was experiencing with Chloe versus my time with Che. I continued to struggle with the fact that Chloe was not the 'same' as other children around her at the same age – and this was most noticeable in terms of family and friends' children. I really struggled with this internally and this increased the sense of inadequacy that would plague me occasionally. I knew that the feelings of self-doubt and guilt were not rational and sensible and were almost like a form of mental self-flagellation. I so wanted

Angels

Chloe to be the 'same' as other children her age and became uncomfortable in settings where we needed to be with other people and their children. On reflection, maybe that was the reason I became distant from some friends. I would often feel like I could not be comfortable managing Chloe's needs and socially interacting. It was such hard work and a lot of unspoken stress that I internalised, so not many people could see that. There was nobody in my social circle who had experienced what I was going through. In fact, autism as a term was not very well understood or even thought about.

It was easier to just keep it simple and make sure we were in settings that I knew would not cause any disruption for those around us or Chloe. I would not have to explain things or answer questions about why Chloe was not speaking much, walking very strongly, or not appearing to be interacting much (the list goes on!). My world became very small and would remain so for a while. Chloe was not automatically invited to birthday parties in my personal circle and not really included – perhaps that was because of my behaviour in trying to manage her needs – but it hurt as I felt some friends did not make the effort either to try to understand and reach out to me to just ask and try to include her. A few did and I will always be grateful for that. This period of my life also started to show me how much effort I made with friendships and when my foot was off the accelerator how much did not happen as a result. The experience was teaching me so much more about my life that was beyond Chloe.

During this time I had to begin the dreaded search for a school as she was due to start in September of the same year. Chloe had found another set of angels at her ASD nursery unit who were also very fond of her. I could see that the team there were committed to the children and passionate about the possibilities and potential in each of them. They helped me understand this world of autism in an educational sense. I learnt how important it was to ensure that Chloe and children like her could 'access' learning and how key it was to start from where they were and understand their world. The nursery head and her team taught me how to accept things that I felt were not 'right' or 'normal' with Chloe. I started to be aware of how 'stimming' – the incessant rocking and flapping of hands – helped to ground and centre Chloe, rather than being some sort of 'issue' that needed to be resolved. Getting this information early in Chloe's development was gold dust. It helped both her dad and me (and Che!) launch into Chloe's world rather than always look at it from our perspectives. We had to unlearn some things, and by doing this we were able to help her in a more effective way and aid her ability to learn and develop.

As a result of Chloe having this positive experience in the ASD nursery unit, I realised how critical it was to ensure that she ended up in the right school placement. Chloe seemed happier with the combination of her childminder, Claire, and the ASD nursery unit team. We established a routine and she had fewer (albeit still very present) meltdowns and was starting to be able to manage situations that previously would have triggered more extreme responses in terms of her emotions and sensory processing needs. Having people around her who understood how to manage her was a critical part of this.

I spent the early part of 2013 looking at a few schools. It was clear to me that a mainstream setting was not going to be right for Chloe, so I focused on specialist provisions – something a year before I would have been hesitant to do but Chloe's needs were determining what was going to be the right path for her. I found one that I thought was the best of a not-so-great bunch and put in the application. It was going to be managed by the local authority special needs department and I waited for confirmation which was due to happen just after the Easter break.

I carried on working as normal and was in the beginning of an expanded remit working globally and establishing a new team with people from all over the world. I had also finally resolved all financial matters relating to my divorce. This stage of the proceedings was particularly painful and extremely stressful. I soldiered on, emboldened by the idea of a virtual finishing line within sight and reach. When it finally arrived I limped over the line, breathed a sigh of relief and scanned the landscape: I was just thankful that this part of my life was finalised and I could work on rebuilding myself.

It was in June 2013, when I came up for air from a very busy work schedule, that I realised I had not received confirmation of Chloe's school placement. What was more concerning was that other children in her nursery unit had. I put a call in to her case worker, who called me back as I was on a lunch dash in between meetings and had the phone to my ear whilst navigating carrying my lunch and purse – a normal experience for me. Her words stopped me dead in my tracks as she said, 'I'm afraid it seems like Chloe did not get a place. I'm really sorry as I'm not sure what has happened here. It looks like we have missed her and I need to find out what has gone wrong.' She paused, waiting for a reaction.

I had stopped just before my building's tall and imposing entrance, stunned into silence. I could not believe what I was hearing. Another failure for my baby girl and another

Angels

fight on the horizon. I did not know how I could respond. The case worker went on to say that she would come back to me. I went back into my office readying myself for another set of letters and campaigning for Chloe as well as a long list of work emails to wade through.

Bodhichitta

The battle to secure a school place for Chloe should never have happened. It was a clear failure on the part of the teams who were there to support Chloe through the school applications process. Nonetheless, I understood that I would need to make sure this was addressed and that Chloe got into the right placement for her. I knew that this would not happen quickly or effectively by just leaving the local authority to address the issue. So I returned to my MP, who had helped me manage the situation with Chloe's exclusion and was familiar with her case. After reviewing what had happened, the MP sent a letter that reminded the respective teams of their responsibilities and that I was now within my rights to commence my own search for a suitable placement, which in this case included the private sector (which if something was found and deemed appropriate for Chloe's needs the local authority would also be obliged to consider and fund).

So another journey commenced to search out the right school placement for Chloe. This was such an important

Bodhichitta

and critical step for her, and I could not afford to get it wrong. I knew the power of Chloe being in the right environment, and had to fight to make sure she landed in the best possible place for her future progress.

At this point I felt as if I was at the bottom of a deep descent. I was emotionally drained and still trying to work through where I was going in my life. I had to pause this self-work for a time and focus completely on the task in hand.

Another lesson I have learnt during the journey with Chloe is the power of focus; laser-like and disciplined. I knew I could achieve the right outcome by remaining clear about the objective as well as being able to deal with curveballs. It was a technique honed from my work, especially when working through complex programmes and having to manage unforeseen events. I also had a natural tendency to be disciplined and focused on achieving, which was something I learnt from observing my parents. They both worked so hard to provide for me and my siblings and never faltered. I admired their tenacity, even through some really challenging times. In my most formative years I had great role models and that was helping me now to be a parent for Chloe. I had determined that Chloe was not going to end up in any school placement, but one that would be right for her.

Bigger Than the Moon

At this point, even though I was at the bottom, shattered and bruised and with no answers, I could see that Chloe was in this place with me, giving me purpose and a reason to keep going and to keep fighting. I felt renewed almost at the point where I felt things had fallen completely apart – when *I* had fallen apart. I discovered strength in the most unexpected way during these moments of despair because of a deep and unconditional love for Chloe, which went beyond being her mother. I felt completely connected to her and my role advocating for her well-being and progress. She was not going to be marginalised because of her disability and I was going to become her warrior, fighting from a place of love. I resolved that I was going to come from that place of love in all my interactions to advocate for Chloe, even with those people that I was angry or frustrated with. The letters and emails would all be titled 'The Plan for Chloe' as with the earlier battle with her nursery. They would first be written from a point of empathy to show that my objective was their objective, and I wrote with kindness, as well as with vulnerability. I was polite, respectful and factual. I wanted all people interacting with this case to not see it as 'just another case' but to know it was about Chloe, a young child who had as much right to the best start as any other child.

Bodhichitta

My network of mums from the EarlyBird NAS parental autism groups were invaluable, and again I especially turned to Natalie. I was learning more and more to be vulnerable and realised there was great strength in doing that as it ensured I was able to get the help needed to achieve my objective. Natalie was always there for me and gave me the names of two schools (both private). One school was a broader specialist provision rather than just ASD specific, however they also supported children on the spectrum who had perhaps a speech and language therapy need, which Chloe did.

I took her to the assessment day full of hope, as always, and when I arrived spoke to the headteacher about Chloe. During the conversation I felt that Chloe was becoming unsettled and I started to have knots in my stomach about what the observation would conclude and whether they thought she would be 'accepted'. All the fears started to come into my mind that she would not fit in and that they could not help her. At this point in the journey I was still battling with this idea of Chloe having to fit in, rather than the environment fitting in with her! I think this was also in some ways a reflection of the work I had to do with myself; accepting who I was and where I was – that would be a longer process. I did not want to have to compromise on getting Chloe into the right environment, despite how desperate the situation was. I still had hope she would end up in the right place. As Chloe got older I would learn that compromise must *never* be an option. It has to be right.

We moved the assessment from the headteacher's office to a class setting with other pupils and that is where it went awry. Chloe became overwhelmed and I guess fearful of where she was and what was happening. Her meltdown began as we tried to get her to take part in an activity; the poor girl just did not know what was happening and the more we pushed the worse it got. I was so stressed and I started to panic internally that this was the end of the world and she would not be accepted anywhere. I could see the look on the teachers' faces and knew that this setting would not be right for Chloe. I left the assessment with Chloe and as soon as we got in the car she instantly calmed down and kept repeating, 'I'm okay now, Mummy.' I felt angry at myself as I believed I'd let her down, again beating myself up unnecessarily.

I called her dad from the car and as usual he listened patiently, reassuring me that it was fine and that we would continue to look at other places. His presence as a co-parent was essential at times like this. I also knew he was firmly in the 'team Chloe' camp and loved her beyond limits, just as I did. My determination to come from a place of love therefore had to apply to him as much as to

Bodhichitta

anyone else; it was probably the most challenging thing I have ever had to do, but I knew if I was guided by the right intention, which was to ensure the well-being of my children, it could never be wrong. However, I would always moderate this with the love I needed to show myself, so there were always boundaries in my interactions with him, especially mentally, and it was a constant balance that had to be managed. My rule was that as long as we were talking about the children and interacting on that basis only, it would be fine as we both loved them in equal measure and were committed to their well-being.

☾

The second assessment was with a relatively new school, and learning from the experience with the previous school, I decided to go there first on my own. As soon as I arrived, I felt like I did when we first met Claire, Chloe's childminder. It was a great place and very calm. The school was completely focused on children with ASD and, importantly for Chloe, the school and its curriculum were geared to ASD children, where learning and progress was expected of the children who went there. The primary school had just been formed and there was one other child who would be starting with Chloe if she was accepted and they would be the inaugural primary class. The environment was well-suited to Chloe as the school was in a semi-rural location; they had animals on site as well as all the therapies that Chloe would need so there would be no need to coordinate bringing people on-site from the various therapy teams (the benefit of being privately funded). I realised that this would also be crucial for Chloe to get this focused and specialised level of support. I had not planned for her to go to a privately funded setting but the standard application process had failed to identify a school place for her and I was not going to fail in my role to make sure this happened.

The school said, as part of the process, they would go and observe Chloe in her current nursery placement. I liked the fact that they wanted to see her in the environment where she was comfortable and would therefore be able to gauge her needs in a way that showed her in her most natural state (even if that meant they observed a meltdown). The headteacher was quick to reassure me that the focus was to make sure they understood Chloe better and ensure they could make an informed decision as to whether they could support her needs and be the right setting for her. This reinforced for me what I had learnt so far in understanding how to help Chloe. I needed to work from her perspective at all times and go from

Bodhichitta

there rather than work her needs around others' perspectives. It's not that I did not believe that Chloe would need to adapt her needs and preferences to certain environments and situations, but that was not going to be the default start point. From now on people needed to first understand her world. If you wanted to be a part of my daughter's life you would need to understand it first and then work back from there.

Chloe was assessed and the report from the school said that they believed they could support her and so offered her a place. It was confirmed with the local authority that they would support the funding required and that brought an intensive month's worth of work and battling to a close – for now. There would be more challenges to experience on the journey with Chloe but I knew that we could overcome them if I remained resilient and focused.

At this stage, I was beginning to realise that there was great joy and fulfilment to be found in times when I probably felt most lost and in despair. The energy received by making your way through 'the wood' when you are, as Dante put it, 'truly lost' is so empowering. It's certainly not easy and I don't want it to ever sound that way; however, I can honestly say that I only began to really know myself and what I was capable of after going through these experiences. Coming out the other side felt like a miracle and

Bigger Than the Moon

in turn I was grateful and appreciative of the process and that I had found a clearing to see something brighter and more hopeful ahead.

Hope is very important for humanity, and for parents of children with special needs it's sometimes all you have when trying to work through issues and ensuring you are doing the very best you can for your child. You always work on the basis of 'What if I am not here?', and whilst this may seem slightly morbid, it is a very practical reality for 'forever parents'. Your child will need you generally more than if they did not have those needs. There is a 'life' dependency. They need you for things like keeping safe, managing their physical needs and keeping them away from situations that may be harmful, especially given their vulnerability, often into adulthood. However, you can't stay in this place of 'what if?' for too long as it affects your ability to manage your own well-being and for you move to onwards. I started to embrace not knowing as much and not being in as much control of my life and leant more on an inner sense of faith and confidence to help guide me to an opening; another door to open to the next place, knowing that it would be okay, eventually.

Instead of transcending the suffering of all creatures, we move toward turbulence and doubt however we can... At the bottom we discover water, the healing water of bodhichitta. Bodhichitta is our heart – our wounded, softened heart. Right down there in the thick of things we discover that love will not die. This love is bodhichitta. It is gentle and warm: it is clear and sharp; it is open and spacious. The awakened heart of bodhichitta is the basic goodness of all beings.

— PEMA CHÖDRÖN,
COMFORTABLE WITH UNCERTAINTY

Labalaba (Butterfly)

The summer before Chloe started school, Susan and I decided to go on another holiday with our children – this time to Disney World in Florida. It had become a bit of an obsession for Chloe, who watched Disney movies and had a Princess Tiana dress. She watched all the clips of Disney World trips people had made on YouTube and was just mesmerised by the idea of this magical place and I wanted her to experience this magic in real life. I was lucky enough to have a best friend who, in her own journey of challenges, understood the importance of ensuring you made the most of every moment and enjoyed life. We both worked really hard and knew to balance that out with some fun and, more importantly, opportunities for self-care. Florida held so many memories for me as a child travelling with my parents. I had also introduced Che to this amazing place of escape. I wanted to mark this next phase of my life and create a new narrative that would be

Labalaba (Butterfly)

for me and the children in this familiar place. I could not think of a better person to do this with than Susan and her son Kyle.

I was now at a point where I felt ready to do the work on myself and really begin to find me again. Until now, I had not been able to properly focus on this as events always seemed to overtake me. I wanted to rediscover that part of myself that had been neglected over the last couple of years and bring some joy back to my life again. I no longer wanted my happiness to rely on someone else or be because of someone else. I just wanted to feel happy because of me. So much of what I had been through illuminated the fact that I had not been anchored. Somewhere along the journey, way before Che and Chloe, I had made the choice (both consciously and unconsciously) to move away from who I was and found myself in other people's worlds. Looking back, this trip with Susan began a process of return to who I was before that decision; a journey that would still be hard and bumpy but was more hopeful.

I wanted to take the opportunity to bring some happiness and fun back to the children's lives as well. I knew that whilst I did my best to shield them from the challenges I was going through personally, they were very much aware of the stress and pressure, and whilst I did my best to manage that, sometimes it would get too much and a tear would fall or I would be sad in front of them. Che was a particularly sensitive child and I wanted to make him feel like the focus for a while. Sharing the world with Chloe was something he loved but I was always aware of the time and energy she required from me and was grateful that he understood and never made me feel as if I was not focusing on him.

We had the best time at Disney World, full of laughter, jokes and stories that will remain with us forever. Susan and I will never forget Chloe being dressed up as Princess Tiana on what had to be the hottest day ever with temperatures reaching the high 90s. Chloe insisted on wearing this dress all day through the heat and the sweat! We could not get her to take it off – it was too hot to battle with her and Chloe's indomitable spirit was not one to play with. I have a picture and video of her staring in wonderment at her surroundings and all the characters, in this huge ballgown dress, watching the traditional show that the characters put on in front of the famous castle. She is singing along with them as they chant 'Dreams do come true' and is focusing intently; it was a moment I will remember forever as I could see that she truly believed it, just like I did when my parents took me to Disney all those years ago, at nearly the same age. I remembered

Labalaba (Butterfly)

that feeling as I watched her feel it too. I have already said that her arrival into this world marked a shift in mine, and this moment helped me to understand why. She not only gave me a purpose, but I felt like she was also going to help me find myself again. She was going to be my guru.

I returned from that holiday renewed and ready to start this next phase of the journey. Chloe started at her new school in the September. Che was also entering his last year of primary school. I was continuing to work at Citi in a global role and travelling intermittently. Coordinating school and work with two children became more complex, which led to a much fuller schedule to manage. There would be school concerts, outings and parents' evenings and, in addition, the other meetings associated with having a child with special needs. These meetings would include things like the annual review process (separate to a standard parent-teacher meeting or end-of-year review), meetings with therapy teachers, reviews when she needed specific help or I'd raised a concern, if I felt something needed to be addressed with her. So I had the usual commitments, as with Che, but with more layers. This required even more coordination with her dad, Che's school and Chloe's childminder. Che's school had a very well-run after-school club; I don't know where I would have been without it. It would have been hard for me to

Bigger Than the Moon

fund a full-time nanny for both of them as I was the sole financial provider for my children.

I also honestly don't know what I would have done without Claire. She was a solid rock for me and never let me down. I knew it was challenging supporting Chloe, and she had other children to look after, but she always provided Chloe with an environment where she could be who she was and also mix with other children who did not have special needs. Claire also knew how to manage Chloe's meltdowns, but I knew it was tough for her making sure it did not disrupt the other children too much. Over time she would learn strategies to pre-empt a meltdown or quickly diffuse it. We both loved Claire and when the time came for Chloe to move on as she transitioned to secondary school, I found it very hard to accept (still do) as I had relied on her more than I realised – not just for Chloe but also for me. We would talk when I picked her up and I could tell her my fears and problems and she would listen without judgement. Parents of children with special needs require this type of support: present but not intrusive. I have also been lucky to have had great support from my sister, who, whilst much younger than me, has been a constant presence and support for both Che and Chloe. She truly is the world's best aunt, who loves them as if they are her own, and

Labalaba (Butterfly)

when I have needed help, she has been there to help me figure things out.

Another person who helped me immensely was Jaime. Jaime was one of the mums at Che's school and her son Freddie and Che became best friends at the school and are connected to this day. I consider him one of my other sons. At my work, Jaime was known amongst my team as Che's 'school mum'. She filled in the gaps I found hard to, given my full-time working schedule. She would tell me about the World Book Days before they happened so I would not forget. She told me about Mufti day and ensured that if there was an after-school activity or outing, I had as much advance notice and a reminder as well. Honestly, she saved me more than once from that disappointed look often seen on children whose parents work full-time, when something has inevitably been forgotten from the class schedule. She also cared for Che as one of her own. He would spend time in her home and with her family, with sleepovers and after-school play dates. As far as I was concerned Jaime worked full-time as a mum of three (later to become four) and also worked part-time. I was always in awe of her organisational skills when it came to managing her life; in some ways we were very much the same – except her profession helped me much more than mine helped hers! I will always be grateful to her for the physical and emotional support she gave to me, Che and Chloe and I hope if she ever reads this she will come to realise how much her presence in my life meant to me and my family. My recommendation to others is to find and seek out your support network and trusted advisors.

Chloe was in her class with one other child, a boy. They had been the first two children in the new primary provision in the school. Chloe's diagnosis of autism at such a young age alerted me to a very stark fact: not many girls were diagnosed early with autism, if at all. I was always the only parent in any group setting whose child was a girl. At first, I thought it was just an anomaly, but then as I became more exposed to different settings and people as part of my autism network, I realised that it was in fact a general trend. I discovered that girls are quite effective at 'masking' the traits typically associated with an autism diagnosis, coupled with the fact that stereotypes also play a part in people misreading or diagnosing traits as other things which are not typically associated with boys, such as being shy or introverted. I believe Chloe's diagnosis happened because I was so focused on addressing the

Labalaba (Butterfly)

feeling I had that something was different about her and my concerns around her development. I also relied more on my intuition that something was not right and refused to listen to platitudes and traditional biases about girls. The system is not necessarily set up to help parents with all of this and so it seems logical that so many girls may be left without support. Parents also may not be aware that they can get more help but it takes a lot to seek it out. There is plenty of research in this space and if you are a parent of a girl with an autism diagnosis or suspect that this may need to be considered, I would encourage you to find out about the research and become informed so you can ensure you are getting the right support for your child.

Most of Chloe's educational life would be in a class of boys, which continues to this day. This never seemed to bother her as she was extremely close with her brother and always around his friends, so she was used to interacting with boys and seemed to be comfortable in their company.

As Chloe was moving into a new stage in her educational life, and learning how to use her wings, I too was on a similar journey in my personal life. She and I would continue to run parallel lives.

Waxing Crescent

Life with Chloe continued to be challenging and beautiful at this stage. Starting school meant learning more about her condition and how it affected her not just from a physical and emotional perspective but now from an academic one. School was a different stage and now we would need to observe how she adjusted in this environment with a broader curriculum, and also how she could engage with it and her level of cognitive understanding. She was learning to fly but it was becoming apparent to me that the way this would happen would not be straightforward or easy and presented more work for me as her parent and advocate. Chloe could read well and this was an area of strength for her. She needed more support with anything related to numbers as this took a little longer for her to grasp conceptually. Her passion was for anything musical; she loved singing and performing and excelled in anything that allowed her to express herself in this way. Chloe had a prodigious memory, which meant that it looked as if she learned quickly but it became apparent that this did not always mean she understood. We had to be very observant along with the school to continuously understand what she was learning and how much of it she was able to process. As her parent, making sure her statement of needs or Educational Health Care Plan (EHCP) was appropriate and reflected what she needed took significant effort.

I had to do a lot of research and get tips from other parents and support organisations on how to navigate the process and ensure Chloe could get the support she needed.

I also came to realise that overcoming one thing was just that. There would be constant things to overcome, deal with, learn about, challenge and fight for. Each time I got over one hurdle I naively thought that would be it. I soon came to realise that this was not the case and talking with other parents of special needs children reinforced that. Over time I recognised that the art would be to accept that and understand that it would always be that way. This understanding grounded and anchored me, so I did not lose focus. Sometimes the reality can be overwhelming, especially when you are dealing with something significant or quite complex. In those times I would say be kind to yourself and try to breathe and stay in the present moment and try not to think too much; I still have to give myself this advice!

There were beautiful moments where Chloe's progress would literally bring tears to my eyes. Her first Christmas concert where she came on stage with her class and teachers to sing is one that stays with me as I knew how challenging and frightening that would have been for her. There was the parents' evening where I would see her exercise books with her writing and how she was starting to form words on the page very deliberately, even if the writing was huge. I also felt proud when she went on her first outing with the school, fully armed with ear defenders and then being proud to tell me she eventually took them off!

Some of the moments would also temper my enthusiasm; her meltdowns were still a big part of her life (and would continue to be) and learning coping strategies and being able to self-regulate would be a big objective in those earlier years and continued as she approached puberty. Learning how to interact with peers continued to be challenging and as in those early days Chloe retreated into her own world and would sometimes appear detached (even though after educational psychologist observations she was found to be very present and very aware in these scenarios). The benefit of being in a specialist

Waxing Crescent

school environment was that you did not have to explain to teachers what was happening. They were equipped with interventions and had good staff ratios to be able to manage. However, it continued to be a very time-intensive process to manage and sometimes took a lot of energy from Chloe. Getting the call before going to pick her up to update on an incident and then her coming home apologising to me – not that she needed to but Chloe always wanted to be seen doing well and the right thing. I saw so much of myself in her. It pained me to see her do the very thing that I was trying to stop myself from doing; beat herself up and self-admonish. I tried to reassure her as much as her little head could comprehend in those days and it is something that I still have to do with her even more as she has got older. Chloe is a brave old soul, and her courage is a big part of why I believe she has managed to progress and develop in school. It was a lesson for me, too, watching her overcome her fears and doubts. She inspired me as I watched and cared for her during those early years, and if I started to feel doubt or fear about anything that was happening in my life, I would think of Chloe and try my hardest to overcome the feeling. It wasn't always smooth sailing but with some practice we established a rhythm and an understanding individually with ourselves and then with each other.

Bigger Than the Moon

In early 2015 my journey took me in a different direction and caused a shift in my personal life. I went on a first date with my now husband. At this stage I believe I felt I was ready to consider starting a new relationship and was very confident about bringing my authentic self to any dating situation. I had done a lot of work to make space for myself and get to know myself better. I was getting more and more comfortable with who I was now and where my life had got to, as opposed to where it had been. I liked who I was and, in a way, had developed a healthy relationship with myself. Because of this, on reflection, whilst meeting him was not planned, it made sense to me that when he did come into my life, it seemed to work. I was not intentionally looking for a life partner, as I had so much else going on in my life. I was also very clear that my children, especially Chloe, were a part of the package and so dating for me was not a 'thing' at this point but I was open to it. From our initial conversations and very first date, talking about our respective children and everything about them was the most natural process. I felt safe around him and there were no concerning questions buzzing round in my head.

As I talked to him about Chloe and her needs, I observed in subsequent dates that he had taken time to learn about autism and he would reference this in conversations with

Waxing Crescent

me way before even meeting Chloe. In every scenario, be it work or personal, being open about Chloe was a very important part of people understanding a critical part of my life that invariably impacted how I showed up to those around me. Creating this level of understanding and awareness is critical. I don't always have the energy or time to keep explaining things and neither do I want to. I just need people to understand and it can't always be my job to make this happen. It is important not to compound the stress of managing autism in your life with concealing it from others. Sharing your story in some ways frees you and allows people to understand who you are and what you have to manage and perhaps be considerate of that. If they are not, well, they do not deserve to be in your life. I would even argue that they can't be.

We would eventually marry, but for this part of the journey over the next few years he became my joy, place of refuge and support. I had arrived at this place of comfort and security and embraced it fully. More importantly, he became a great support for my children, which for me was everything. He had to learn this world of autism too and probably showed up at a very challenging stage in both my children's lives. Chloe would encounter a number of difficulties as the COVID pandemic and lockdowns hit, and Che was a young boy about to enter adolescence,

Bigger Than the Moon

so no easy time. His children had become adults by the time he met me, so entering back into the tunnel was not something I imagined that he thought he would be doing and certainly not one that looked like this – but enter he did and he has supported us all the way as we have travelled through the twists and turns.

He also helped me to see beyond Chloe's perceived 'limitations' and from day one recognised the potential in her when sometimes I had got into a habit of compensating for her needs and perhaps thinking of things she couldn't do rather than what she could do. It's so easy to get into habits when you are the parent of a special needs child having to do more for them than in a typical situation, and he helped me with seeing how Chloe could be more independent and self-sufficient. I think by coming into her life when he did, he was not bogged down by the last few years of pre- and early diagnosis. His view was more present and forward-looking, so he was able to open my mind up to other possibilities I may have been too tired to see at that point.

He is also a talented pianist and he introduced me to a certain method of learning the piano – the Suzuki method (his daughter had learned this way as well.) We had a beautiful piano at home that I dabbled playing with now and again and I felt like its purpose was somehow

Waxing Crescent

linked to Chloe. Suzuki method focuses primarily on helping children to learn first through listening and children normally commence lessons at three years old. By this stage Chloe was eight.

One evening, quite late, as I was surfing the internet I typed in 'Suzuki method tutors near me' and stumbled across a tutor online who happened to be located very near to me. Her name was Eleanor, and not thinking too much I dropped a note to her website telling her about Chloe and explaining that she was autistic but with a love of music and a prodigious memory and I believed she had the potential to learn piano.

I was not even sure Eleanor would respond, and if the truth be known I was also a bit hesitant about it all, thinking that having goals like this for Chloe was a bit of a stretch. Just getting her to navigate the foundations of learning at school and to self-regulate were big goals and I wondered if this was beyond her current potential. But a day later a lovely email came back to me. Again, it was the same feeling I had when all the other people who have helped Chloe came into our lives; her tone was warm and open, ready to explore the idea, and when I got over my initial nerves I sensed that this person was going to at least be curious to explore if she could support Chloe. My instincts told me to keep going and meet her to find out more. What a beautiful journey that would turn out to be. Eleanor became her tutor and in a funny way, like her childminder, Claire, her friend. Chloe and I love her and through her talent, I have learnt so much observing Eleanor's lessons with Chloe: the art of patience, of taking steps and taking them again. Most of all I have learnt through the music lessons about not giving up: watching Chloe progress through early stages of learning with one finger and very basic notes I would have my stomach in knots thinking it would not work out. But I was calmed by Eleanor's quiet confidence and her clear conviction that this was a 'years' process not a 'months' one. She also saw Chloe's unique gifts as advantages (and focused less on the autism). So things like her ability to remember and learn quickly through sound and to engage with the music and intuitively learn effectively were evident to Eleanor and she worked from this perspective rather than from any perceived disadvantage.

Chloe's ability to focus intently was a big part of her being able to learn the piano technique; her concentration was above normal, especially for a child of her age. Of course Eleanor recognised accessing Chloe's ability to understand and comprehend concepts needed some care and thought, as well as patience, such as how to work with Chloe's processing speed, which could be

Waxing Crescent

much slower for some aspects of learning and faster for others. Chloe would not always get things right and she would sometimes get frustrated very quickly. She could not learn music theory as easily, so Eleanor would naturally work with her from where she was and go from there, either drawing pictures or using materials, toys and simulation games. Over time, as Chloe's fluency and confidence increased in her playing, I too would be more relaxed and grateful that I decided to be brave and reach out to Eleanor with that email, not expecting much of a reply but in the end receiving more than I could imagine.

☾

This period would see a number of 'firsts' for Chloe. Her first time going to a bowling alley is etched in my mind. Bowling was something we had loved to do as a family and it was my sincerest wish that this could continue with Chloe. The noises of a bowling alley, the echo and slam of the skittles as they get knocked down and the screams and cheers of people not only in the alley but in the games arcade all made this a fearful process for her and me, but again preparation was key. Talking to Chloe about what she may experience, letting her watch YouTube videos of bowling alleys and just being confident and excited about

Bigger Than the Moon

the prospect of her first bowling experience, made her want to go and confront any fears. The moment we were able to take her to the metal frame that assists young children to aim for a strike without having to lift the ball was priceless: I have a picture of her looking very happy with herself and her brother equally happy for her.

Another first was going to the cinema. This was possibly one of my most nervous moments with her as the cinema presented a number of sensory processing challenges; the darkness of the environment, the surround sound effects and unexpected special effects during a film all made for the potential of a significant meltdown. Taking this chance in a cinema where people go to watch a film without wanting to be disturbed was a risk. The cinema chain we went to offered autism-friendly screenings and I sat down with her one day and explained we could go to that. I told her the lights would be dimmed so not completely dark, and the sound turned down. She looked at me intently for a while and her mind was clearly processing something. After a few minutes of quiet thinking, she said very clearly that she wanted to go to the normal showing of the film like 'my brother goes to' and insisted that Che come along with us. It's like she became the buffalo about to confront the storm, and off we three went to see *Sing*. I knew she was scared but I also knew she wanted to be brave. She sat between me and Che. We looked at her as the trailers commenced and I hugged her tight as the Dolby surround sound ad came on with pulsating speakers and echoes all round. She clung to me tightly and just put her hands over her ears and her head into my chest. Once the ad was over she sat back and smiled; a look of satisfaction came over her and we all enjoyed the film. The joy of watching her laugh and just be in the moment moved me beyond words. No words can describe the seemingly small steps that are giant leaps in the world of autism.

There are so many things I continue to learn being a parent on this journey with autism. There are the highs and lows, as well as coming to terms with the fact that this is a different journey to the one that I had planned for my life. I have had to work really hard to accept that truth; acceptance has been the hardest thing to navigate and come to terms with. In one of my blog posts I reflect on this uncomfortable truth:

> How often, in moments of challenge, uncertainty and most likely battling tiredness, do we say to ourselves 'Why me?' and 'I wish things had been different?' Some people struggle to admit this to themselves and others, but I never have. I believe

that it is at these moments, when those feelings of regret arrive, we meet our ally 'Acceptance'.

Some of us meet Acceptance and choose not to acknowledge its presence. I feel this is most often due to a fear that by doing this you may not be moving forward or you are accepting that things may never change. However, in my journey with Chloe and with life in general, it's been essential to embrace the need to accept that some things are just the way they are and the ability to move forward comes from evolving how you manage and deal with that.

I end the post by saying,

Moving forward is essential for human progress and evolution, however it is important to be kind to yourself in the process and not prevent yourself from feeling what you feel. Acceptance can ensure you don't stay in that feeling; that you face it, even embrace it, and then move on taking one step at a time.

Waxing Crescent

For those of you on a similar journey – or perhaps even those going through a challenging time of a different nature – I hope that by sharing my experience it can, in some way, help you as you go through your journey and find your way to that open door. So much is waiting for you.

The Beginning

When I let go of what I am, I become what I might be.

— LAO TZU

From my Blog *'Bigger Than the Moon'* (16 June 2019)

Be Still: Closing the door to Time

> 'I wish it need not have happened in my time,' said Frodo. 'So do I,' said Gandalf, 'and so do all who live to see such times. But that is not for them to decide. All we have to decide is what to do with the time that is given us.
>
> — J. R. R. Tolkien, *The Fellowship of The Ring*

Time is such an elusive concept; just when we think we have dimensioned it and put it into a neat box of calendars, of appointments, of schedules, it turns around and knocks us out with something we did not count on or plan for. Then our perception shifts, depending on what has happened: time may slow right down and force us to be completely still, in other cases it completely speeds up and we are left in a tailspin trying to understand what is happening and how

The Beginning

to get back to neutral again, to a normal pace of time – whatever that looks like.

A recent conversation with Chloe's piano tutor is the reason I find myself pondering on time. We are talking about octaves and going through scale practice with Chloe. The Suzuki method of teaching piano is heavily concentrated on being able to listen and hear the notes, rhythms and pulses. Chloe is intuitively able to understand music concepts and theory and it is clearly one of her strengths. She talks to Chloe about what an octave is and what kind of shape an octagon is – how many sides does it have and so on – until she gets to the figure eight. Eight notes in an octave. We then get into a history of the number eight and talk about what the month October means then if it is the tenth month in the year – as often happens between her tutor and I with our naturally inquisitive thirst for all interesting facts!

She tells me that at one point there were only ten months in the calendar year and we discuss the changes and shifts in how history and the people in it have measured time and how manufactured a concept it is, depending on what has happened and when in the world order.

Bigger Than the Moon

October was originally the eighth month of the Roman calendar. It comes from the Latin word 'octo' meaning eight. Then it became the tenth month when January and February were added to the calendar. Julius Caesar made this change for detailed reasons I will not go into for this blog, but safe to say time has not always been the way it is today.

So you may ask why am I writing about this? As I reflect on my experience with autism, I realise how much it has altered my perception of time. In the early days pre-diagnosis it sped time up. I am finding it hard to recall all the moments of those early years and write them down for the book – of how hard it was, and how sleep-deprived I became and having to go to work every day like the world was normal. Showing up for meetings and presentations having had very little sleep the night before, of picking my daughter up at her nursery and seeing her distressed as she struggled to manage her meltdowns and became the target of a lot of parents' ignorance of the fact that some children are just not made the same. Of the days going to appointments and seeing doctors all the while trying to hold myself

The Beginning

together and just to have the goal to be able to get up in the morning. Of not having much time to be with friends and socialise because my energy was so spent. Time went by so quickly and maybe my mind just moved on in order to forget.

Then came the magic of time slowing down. The moment when reality hits you; when you know what you are dealing with and you decide to face it, head on. Those years I can recall with such clarity. It is so clear: the wonderful holidays with my best friend and her son, sitting with Chloe and just watching her be in the world and seeing how great her brother was with her. Being still in the meltdowns and having strategies to manage it which mainly focused on blocking the man-made world out and letting the natural one in. Being where time stood still. All the great meditations and yogic practices target that place of stillness. It is where you find a peace; a place where time does not really exist. You just are.

In the moments I have not been still, I have sometimes slipped into self-pity – and asked why this had to happen to me? What can I do to fix it? But the better moments have been where

Bigger Than the Moon

> I have been still and decided what to do with the things that life has presented to me. Like finding Chloe's piano tutor and sending her a random email to see if she would be remotely interested in teaching a child on the spectrum and getting her response that she would love to talk to me about it. Meeting her and finding a person with such openness and warmth who took Chloe in and helped bring out her gift and who provides me with many beautiful moments on a Saturday morning listening to them both play and sing.
>
> I have learnt to try not to watch time or question what has happened but just be where I am and as Gandalf says, 'Decide what to do with the time that is given us.'
>
> I decided to accept and find out what was possible for Chloe and also for me in this journey and so far we have learnt and done some amazing things.

Taken from my journal, October 2015 – trip to Abu Dhabi

Travelling with my two adorable but very challenging children, Che and Chloe, I felt the need to jot down some thoughts. Chloe has autism. A condition that at once moves and frustrates me. Time with Chloe is often a see-saw between moments of joyous ecstasy and a quiet sadness, sometimes even anger. She has taught me so much about myself and the capacity of the human spirit. When you want, you can achieve amazing things both for yourself and those around you. Time with Chloe is never dull, and I do have to be careful not to expect too much understanding from my wonderful son Che – although he always continues to surprise me with his innate sense of knowledge of his sister's behaviour, language and frustrations. It is a challenge for any sibling of an autistic child to feel visible as they can often disappear amidst all the focus that can sometimes be required for the child affected by autism. As parents we must never lose sight of this. You just work very hard to create some space for the other child to just 'be'. My approach has been to work with

Bigger Than the Moon

Chloe first, so that everything and everybody else can also get seen to with as little disturbance as possible. It's often a guilt-ridden job but I accept it completely, out of pure unconditional love.

Navigating the airport, as with everything around Chloe, is a strategy: a well-timed and well-planned execution of exquisite precision. I have always set myself an ambitious task of travelling with both my children since they were very young babies. It's especially ambitious when one of those children has autism. Chloe's autism affects her in a number of ways – but changes to routine and sudden differences in a schedule are the things that trouble her the most, and very loud, sudden noises, bangs, lights and lots of people around can sometimes have the most profound effect on her and at other times she zones out so much to the extent they have no effect on her at all.

It makes planning a holiday for Chloe a mammoth task. This time I calculate a six-hour flight to the UAE should be manageable. We have done nine hours now four times the other way across the Atlantic Ocean to the Caribbean and the US. Although she was much younger then, the challenges on one hand seemed far more intense, but from another perspective they also were simpler given how young she was. There have been advantages and disadvantages as she has gotten older. Before we could

The Beginning

navigate her physical mobility (and need to wander off and explore) with the control of the 'buggy'. Disadvantage: cumbersome and requiring the strength of a WWE fighter to first get her in and then to strap her in. The usual body contortions of a child Chloe's age (at the time) become even more intense with the strength and voraciousness of a meltdown. I have learnt the art of zoning out and being aware of only myself and Chloe. For me, this is the only way to ensure that any period of a meltdown is managed very quickly and effectively. If you are calm and still, eventually they become calm and still. If you let frustration take over and your awareness of everyone's stares, it quickly deteriorates into something harder to control.

As we walk through the airport on this occasion to see my sister in Abu Dhabi, Chloe is six years old and possessed with such a forceful nature (making it hard to discern what may be triggered from her autism and what may just be her!) – it is hard to tell her what to do and focus her attention. She wants to walk around; she wants to explore and navigate her senses around all the noises and things she is seeing. Chloe's sensory challenges mean she is stimulated by sounds and light more than your neurotypical child at this age. At the time I did not understand this as much as I do now. Now I fully understand

Bigger Than the Moon

why Chloe may zone out, why she may decide to shut her attention off to me and those around her and almost seem lost in the world. Now I realise that it may be us who are lost; Chloe is wide awake. It's a feeling I have as I look at her; depending on what sense has been awoken, she is either intently listening, observing, feeling, touching and trying to connect and understand at a level I believe it is hard for any of us to understand. So whilst it looks like she may have zoned out, I see now that she is actually zoning in. At the time of this trip however I am still evolving my understanding of Chloe's world so am just completely overtaken with the job of staying with her – and trying to make sure she is not too disruptive! What makes situations like this recover from complete desperation to a sense of feeling rescued is the understanding of another person. This time it is a flight attendant who looks like she understands. Us autism parents know that look when others recognise that we need some help; it is without judgement and a need to know the details of the situation and it's just about wanting to help. She reaches over to Chloe from the barrier that is up to stop passengers from boarding and smiles and starts talking to her. Chloe stops and looks up at her with an equally knowing gaze. This gaze is typical when Chloe intuitively connects with someone who has connected with her and understands.

The Beginning

The flight attendant comes over to me and discreetly says she can get me to board as a priority if I need assistance. I absolutely take her up on the offer. Another lesson I have learnt on this journey: I have had to make myself feel comfortable in the world of vulnerability and be ready to know where I actually need help. This is very hard for me but this whole experience with autism has meant that I have no choice if I am to work through the challenges and move forward.

Onward.

Epilogue

I am at peace. I feel like who I am and who I have been trying to find all this time. At time of writing this, a number of years have passed. Where I left the story in 2017 is not the end by any means; there have been many more challenges we have had to work through: transition to secondary school in the middle of a global pandemic, Chloe's father falling seriously ill just as the pandemic hit as well as further battles. The journey continues, and perhaps this is for another book at another time.

It feels like the decade that has passed, where everything changed for me, has been one of renewal and discovery and a time to find strength in a way I never thought possible. I am writing these words listening to the whistling frog whistle in the trees on a warm night in the Caribbean. The familiar sound is a persistent backdrop to me writing these words and signals the setting of the sun in one sense but also that its light will continue to shine on the side of the moon's surface that we see. I realise that both the sun and the moon are ever present and never

Epilogue

really go anywhere. At once mutually exclusive and interdependent – they work together and co-exist to ensure the world keeps turning and providing energy for all who occupy her. They are a constant power illuminating the way for all of us on this amazing planet. I am reflecting how blessed and lucky I feel to have come through my journey of the last ten years and to find myself in this beautiful place. It feels as if it has been a journey of good and bad. I realise now, observing the sun and the moon interplay with each other, that opposites work together towards a common outcome. I believe all the things that happen to us, both good and bad, are necessary to bring something together – to join up and not take apart. The work we have to do to help this process, is figuring that out. We have to try hard to dig deep and ride the waves of uncertainty – sometimes trauma – and keep a form of faith (whatever your belief) that it will all work out: my journey with Chloe and autism has taught me that.

I don't know what is next and I don't need to know. I have concluded that the greatest achievement in any journey is to have discovered something more about who you are and your purpose. As for the rest – what will be will be.

Lessons and Learning

- Get to know who you are and build up your emotional and physical strength – you are your child's greatest advocate and opportunity.
- There were many lessons I believe I personally had to learn from my experience with Chloe, and one of the most important is the art of listening; truly listen to yourself and others.
- My guidance to anyone who is navigating the world of diagnosis for someone they care for, or in any time of immense change, whatever the situation, is to really embrace vulnerability. Be clear and honest with yourself first about what you need so that you can try to get the support that may be required. Being strong may require you to be weak for a while as you try to adjust to what is happening.
- Lean into your intuition not away from it.

Bigger Than the Moon

- Learn the importance of taking moments to stop and be in silence.
- Advocacy for your child must also come from other sources and not just yourself; whilst you are the best one, you need others to join you in order to get the best support for your child – be relentless in seeking out your co-advocates.
- The power of letting go is immense.
- If you are working during these moments of transition, try to be brave and find people at work you can confide in, who can provide you with the space to be able to keep going.
- Become the buffalo (See Chapter 'Buffalo' page 76).
- Be kind to yourself always. The process of discovery is as much about you as it is about the child. You will have to learn how to deal with the present and worry less about the 'whys' and 'ifs' of the past. The help that is needed at diagnosis and discovery is how to move forward and less about how you got there.
- Have a plan. It is important to ensure you raise matters quickly, urgently and in parallel. Don't sit and wait and think the system is going to automatically help you.

Lessons and Learning

- There is only so much 'self-care' work you can do on your own!
- Don't always accept what you hear the first time and seek help where you need to. If you don't know how to do this, seek out those who do. Contact your local MP, Citizens Advice Bureau (if in the UK or the equivalent in your country) and if you have the means, speak to a law firm specialising in SEN.
- Your mindset is extremely important: always ask yourself 'What's the upside?'
- Mastering your ego is a continuous process. Learning to be brave and bold when you don't have the answers is so important.
- Siblings of children with special needs also require as much attention.
- Hope is very important for humanity and for parents of children with special needs. It's sometimes all you have when trying to work through issues and ensuring you are doing the very best you can for your child.
- If you are a parent of a girl with an autism diagnosis or suspect that this may be needed I encourage you to find out about the research on the difference between rates of diagnosis between

genders and become informed, so you can then ensure you are getting the right support for your child.

- Sometimes this reality can be overwhelming, especially when you are dealing with something significant or quite complex. In those times be kind to yourself and try to breathe and stay in the present moment and try not think too much.
- It's important not to compound the stress of managing autism in your life with somehow concealing it from others. Sharing your story in some ways frees you and allows people to understand who you are and what you have to manage and perhaps be considerate of that.

Acknowledgements

I have to thank my tribe and Chloe's tribe. The people who have walked this part of the journey with us and many of them continue to do so. Although there were times I often felt very alone, I never really was.

Mum and Dad – for providing me with such a solid foundation built on unconditional love, resilience, tenacity and hard work. You are my role models and have helped me to be the parent I am today.

My sister Simone, thank you for being there, it is appreciated more than you know. What a gift for my children to have you as their aunt! To my brother Nathan for understanding Chloe's world and helping me to navigate the world of special needs with your expertise.

Susan, Chloe's first true friend and my bestie for life. No words can describe how your presence in my life and my children's lives has enriched us and provided a constant safe harbour. Thank you.

I am thankful for co-parenting: I believe my children have benefited greatly from this.

Bigger Than the Moon

To my grandmother: I know you have been walking with me in this earthly journey from another plane/dimension. I wish you could have met Chloe, but I know your spirit travels through her. I hope you can see that the generational cycle has been broken; mother-daughter love is whole again.

Natalie, who I first met at an EarlyBird NAS parenting support group, and in whom I recognised a fellow warrior! Thank you for being on the other end of a phone or WhatsApp. Your friendship, guidance, support and advice has helped me more than you know: I thank you and appreciate you.

Chloe's childminder, into whose arms she lovingly fell after the challenges with her private nursery and who cared for Chloe from 2013 to 2021 and with whom we are still connected to this day.

Eleanor, Chloe's Suzuki piano teacher, who answered my random email to see if she would be open to teaching an autistic child piano, and brought a talent to life in Chloe, as well as friendship.

Chloe's fabulous, amazing and devoted teachers who were a part of the early years of her educational journey. The fight was worth it for Chloe to have access to the right learning environment and I am grateful for their time and attention.

Acknowledgements

Meghan, thank you for always being there and for including Chloe in moments where many might forget her.

My friends and colleagues who supported mine and Chloe's journey in those early years (even if you did not realise it) – Tamika Niles, Michelle Watkins, Michelle Stubbs, Jackie Ferguson, Cheryl (Chezah) Cummings, Brian Messam, Courtney Phinn, Lisa Forrest, Meghan Cannarella-Harrison, Jaime Griffiths, Russ Kumar, Eddie Ahmed, Susan Catalano, Jackie Fasitta (and the whole Fasitta clan!), Tuyanne Mah-Lee, Alim A. Dhanji, Rebecca Ariyo, Gaynor Nightingale, Claire Miller, Daryl King, Gemma Lines, Anna Collins, James Mendes, Janie Deignan, Dawn Thomas, Junior Green, Joy Miller – thank you.

My many work colleagues across the years and across the world from America to Asia and everywhere in between – thank you.

To those whose friendships I had during this time and who supported me but then became lost for one reason or another; I want to thank you too, as you played an important part in this journey also.

I have been privileged and lucky to be able to write this book at home in the UK and in many other parts of the world which inspired me immensely. Special mention to my second home city, New York – in a way it started with you. Tobago, Barbados, Florida, Abu Dhabi and my island Jamaica. The first draft of this book was finished in Port Antonio, Jamaica.

The first step to making it a reality for publishing was because of a conversation with Julia Hobsbawm, who fired up the process and became an invaluable guide throughout. Thank you, Julia.

Thank you to all the team at Whitefox Publishing for believing in my story and the journey I wanted to share, in order to help someone else. The editing process was very new for me and another moment for me to learn. Thank you Jonathan Eyers for understanding what I was trying to do and working with me to make sure the reader could see that too. Thank you also to Jill Sawyer for making sure it was just right (even when I thought it had all been done!). Sarah Rouse – thank you for your patience as I juggled this project with all the other things happening in my very busy life.

My love of literature started with my mum and her introducing me to reading books way before I even started school and my world became so much richer as a result. This account of my journey has been inspired, assisted, supported and guided by the words of others who I have acknowledged but I want to give a special mention to the

Acknowledgements

following people, without whom I would have remained truly lost. Toni Morrison – I first met you in 1994 in *The Bluest Eye* and never let you go. Thank you for your art and for inspiring me to recount my journey with Chloe with the words, *'If there's a book that you want to read, but it hasn't been written yet, then you must write it.'* Maya Angelou: my constant companion. Ram Dass and Pema Chödrön, for helping me understand myself better. Richard Wright and Ralph Ellison, for helping me to put words on a page confidently, authentically and in a way that only conveyed the truth. Lao Tzu: I found you right at the bottom and your words lifted me to a new way of thinking. I was introduced to Dr Clarissa Pinkola Estes and her seminal work, *Women Who Run With Wolves*, by Karla Gahan (thank you, Karla!): there are truly no words to describe the arrival of her work into my life and the impact it had on my ability to not only write this book but recognise and articulate some of the experiences, learning and feelings I went through in the process. What a gift this work is to the world, and I hope my story introduces more people to her art and wisdom: thank you for being a part of my arrival to 'Bodhichitta'.

And the last thanks goes to my love, my husband, Boyowa. There are no words to express how blessed I feel

Bigger Than the Moon

to have you as a part of my life and this stage of my journey. This book would not have been written and come to life if it were not for your belief in me and the journey. You push me higher and we go together.

To my loyal and faithful companion, Indigo. You were by my side for all of this journey and beyond. The love of a pet is immeasurable and irreplaceable. I will never forget you. Sunset, 25/11/24.

The Moon does not fight. It attacks no one. It does not worry. It does not try to crush others. It keeps to its course, but by its very nature, it gently influences. What other body could pull an entire ocean from shore to shore? The Moon's faithful to its nature and its power is never diminished.

— MING-DAO DENG

www.ingramcontent.com/pod-product-compliance
Ingram Content Group UK Ltd.
Pitfield, Milton Keynes, MK11 3LW, UK
UKHW020205130325
4975UKWH00010B/98